Practical Uveitis
Understanding the Grape

Practical Uveitis
Understanding the Grape

Gwyn Samuel Williams

Consultant Ophthalmic Surgeon, Singleton Hospital, Abertawe
Bro Morgannwg University Health Board, Swansea

Mark Westcott

Consultant Ophthalmic Surgeon, Moorfields Eye Hospital, London
Consultant Ophthalmic Surgeon, Barts Heath, London
Honorary Senior Lecturer, UCL Institute of Ophthalmology, London

Foreword by Carlos Pavesio
Illustrated by Bushra Thajudeen

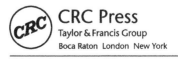

CRC Press
Taylor & Francis Group
Boca Raton London New York

CRC Press is an imprint of the
Taylor & Francis Group, an **informa** business

CRC Press
Taylor & Francis Group
6000 Broken Sound Parkway NW, Suite 300
Boca Raton, FL 33487-2742

Printed in Canada by Webcom Inc.

International Standard Book Number-13: 978-1-138-03575-1 (Paperback)
978-1-138-30369-0 (Hardback)

Visit the Taylor & Francis Web site at
http://www.taylorandfrancis.com

and the CRC Press Web site at
http://www.crcpress.com

Contents

Foreword

The authors start their introduction stating that 'Few subjects terrify ophthalmologists in training more than uveitis', which I think encapsulates a widespread view about this subject, especially amongst trainees, but also by many senior ophthalmologists who share this view when confronted with a patient presenting with visual reduction due to an inflammatory condition. Many large text books are available, which are very complete and up-to-date, but may be quite difficult to use on a day-to-day basis when you are in front of a patient with uveitis and need help to decide what to do.

Practical Uveitis: Understanding the Grape is a book designed to tackle this problem and to allow clinicians to make sense of the clinical signs and organise their thinking regarding type of uveitis, severity, investigations that may be helpful and those that may be unnecessary, or even generate confusion, and how best to manage the different presentations.

The book starts with the necessary basic concepts and cleverly explores the classification of uveitis as an important element for the following steps. The correct recognition of the site of primary involvement, which can only be defined following thorough examination of the anterior and posterior segment, is essential for the elaboration of a differential diagnosis list and for the decisions about what other information will be necessary to achieve the final diagnosis and establish your treatment strategy.

Subsequent chapters deal with the different anatomic sites affected with uveitis and cover all the key aspects of the clinical presentations, critical use of tests and many of the pitfalls related to incorrect interpretation of findings and scattered approach to testing. The rationale for the questioning of patients about other general health problems and request of investigations is well explained and will immensely help those with less experience in this field. They also, very clearly, go over the rationale for the introduction of therapy, especially when and how to start and how to monitor and taper. They present a very broad discussion on posterior uveitis, which represents the most worrying form when it comes to visual loss and importantly, they address the issue of the sight-threatening uveitis, expanding on the most common and aggressive conditions. There is a very good discussion on vascular involvement, a subject which many times confuses even experienced uveitis specialists.

A dedicated chapter to episcleritis and scleritis summarises these important inflammatory conditions, which can, in many cases, be associated with a severe systemic disease that may result in significant health issues if not quickly recognised and managed.

The final chapters deal with the use of immunosuppressive therapy and new developments in the management of uveitis. There is a good overview of the various alternatives, the indication for their use and the dangers associated with their use, apart from the always worrying issue of use of drugs in pregnancy. The new alternatives include a good description of the use of biologics, which are becoming increasingly more used.

This book is loaded with pearls and the tables and illustrations will undoubtedly be a great asset to all those who want to be able to confront a patient with uveitis with more confidence

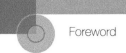

and will help them structure their thinking and make adequate use of investigations and make a well-balanced assessment of the available information to reach the right decision regarding diagnosis and management.

I congratulate the authors on this achievement. This a balanced and clear text on a difficult topic.

Carlos Pavesio

Acknowledgement

Many thanks to Sandrine Westcott for her heroic efforts in proofreading the text.

Authors

Gwyn Samuel Williams qualified from a medical school at King's College London and completed his ophthalmology training on the Wales circuit. He recently completed a year's fellowship in medical retina and uveitis at Moorfields Eye Hospital in London. From June 2016 onwards he has been a consultant in Swansea specialising in medical retina and inflammatory eye disease. He has a keen interest in reading, writing and hiking through the beautiful Welsh countryside.

Mark Westcott is a consultant ophthalmologist at Moorfields Eye Hospital, where he specialises in uveitis, and at St Bartholomew's and The Royal London Hospitals in London. After residency training in London he spent a Fellowship year in glaucoma at the UCLA Stein Eye Institute, Los Angeles. Thereafter, he returned to Moorfields Eye Hospital to undertake a Specialist Fellowship in medical retina and inflammatory eye disease. Mark has co-authored over 40 scientific papers, and regularly lectures both nationally and internationally. He is an honorary senior lecturer at the Institute of Ophthalmology, UCL. His research interests include infectious uveitis, birdshot disease and visual dysfunction in glaucoma. Mark lives in London with his family, and in his spare time he indulges in a passion for amateur astronomy and coaches junior rugby.

Introduction

Few subjects terrify ophthalmologists in training more than uveitis. Along with paediatric ophthalmology and strabismus it represents a seemingly closed box of thought that is all but impenetrable to the non-specialist. The heady combination of rapidly blinding conditions mixed in with benign conditions, of potentially fatal immunosuppressant medication used to control inflammation and specialist nomenclature used to describe phenomena that are not used anywhere else in ophthalmology can turn many junior ophthalmologists away from the field of ocular inflammation. Uveitis specialists are few and far between and unless schooled in the language of inflammation can appear to the uninitiated to be akin to alchemists, seemingly diagnosing and treating conditions based on their own knowledge and experience without a framework to work from. It is almost as if the bottom few rungs of the ladder are missing in uveitis training.

This is a great shame as ocular inflammation is one of the most interesting areas of ophthalmology. It is the most medical of the sub-specialties, and a working knowledge of rheumatology, microbiology and immunology helps immeasurably. Liaising with specialists in other branches of medicine is a common event in the uveitis clinic, and whereas most ophthalmologists look inward at their own discipline the uveitis specialist looks out of the window at the beautiful view outside and can see patterns that join their street, their building, with those around them. Patients if treated correctly can be saved from blindness and even death. The conditions are immensely interesting and once the inflammation has been brought under control the tasks of keeping the immune system under control, defeating infection and dealing with the after-effects of ocular damage require an active use of medical knowledge and make each patient encounter an intellectually satisfying experience. This book aims to make the field of uveitis more accessible by providing a simple framework by which to understand the basics and provide those bottom few rungs to the ladder that seem to be missing.

Many great books have been written about ocular inflammation – encyclopaedic texts and very thorough books containing all the most up-to-date information you would ever be likely to wish for. I have had great textbooks with me in clinic but when faced with a new and frightening situation such as a patient with panuveitis those books, without prior knowledge, might not be so helpful in calming your nerves and telling you what to do. This book aims to provide that much-needed basic knowledge structured in such a way that it is possible to look up a condition such as 'intermediate uveitis' and be guided: What questions to ask, what tests to order and what treatment to deploy.

For example, what does 'uveitis' mean? This question was asked in the all-Wales ophthalmic Christmas quiz a few years ago and very few people knew. Do you know? It is derived from the Latin word for grape, 'uva', hence the title of this book. If the scleral covering of the eye is peeled away the uveal tract underneath resembles a black grape. The suffix '-itis' denotes inflammation. The pictures in this book are sketches of eyes and not the glossy colour pictures you will find in the large uveitis tracts. The purpose of this is to draw the reader's attention to the salient features that differentiate one condition from another and are akin to an Ordnance Survey map rather than Google Earth. At the end of the day people are more likely to use a map

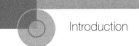

than Google Earth when planning a route, though the latter provides far more actual detail of the terrain once a destination is reached.

Hopefully this increased understanding will generate interest and further information in more detailed textbooks will then be made accessible. If a non-uveitis specialist reads this book and when faced with a patient in eye casualty with an inflammatory eye condition they have never previously seen or heard of gladly accepts the challenge then writing this book will have been worth the effort.

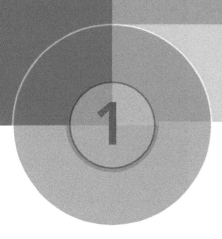

Classification of uveitis

The classification of uveitis is paramount to its understanding. Working out what is the cause of the disease, and hence how to treat it, is dependent on being able to classify it. Uveitis, inflammation of a portion or all of the uveal tract, can be classified according to the anatomical location of the inflammation, the severity and the course of the disease, and the cause of the uveitis. Classifying by cause is not so useful when seeing a patient for the first time and will not be discussed in detail here. Classifying by severity and course is useful but by far the most vital part of approaching a patient with inflammatory eye disease is knowing where the primary site of the inflammation is located, and whether one or both eyes are involved.

CLASSIFICATION BY ANATOMICAL LOCATION

When a patient with an inflamed eye enters eye casualty the main filter that will guide you in diagnosing and treating the problem is the anatomical location of the primary site of the inflammation. The uveal tract, a highly vascularised pigmented layer of tissue located between the retina on the inside and the sclera on the outside, is split into three main parts (Figure 1.1). These consist of the iris anteriorly, the ciliary body immediately behind this forming a band 6 mm wide posterior to the iris root, with everything behind this forming the choroid.

The inflammation may be primarily located in the iris, in which case the condition is called anterior uveitis, the ciliary body and vitreous, in which case the condition is called intermediate uveitis, or any 'back of the eye structure' such as the retina, retinal vessels or choroid, in which case posterior uveitis is the term. If all three are inflamed and it is not really possible to tell if one location is worse than any other then panuveitis is the term. Human tissue rarely gets inflamed in isolation of course and if one location is inflamed then it is common for surrounding tissues to be involved to a greater or lesser degree, in which case knowing which is the primary or most severely involved site is key. Anterior uveitis, for example, can spill over to the ciliary body and anterior vitreous to an extent although the signs are worse anteriorly. Likewise intermediate uveitis can have signs anteriorly and posteriorly as well so looking where the signs are most severe is time well spent in clinic and not doing this properly can lead to diagnostic errors. A fire in one building on a street can result in smoke pouring from not only the building on fire but some smoke escaping from those structures next door as well. Knowing where the smoke is densest will guide firefighters to where to direct their hoses and spraying all buildings without thought to where the main fire is will result in unnecessary water damage and delay in extinguishing the fire.

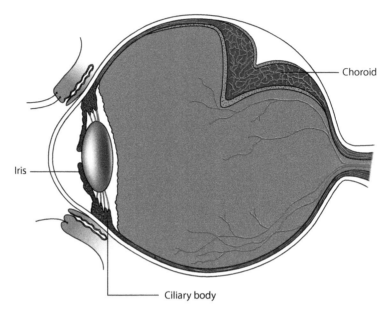

Choroid

Iris

Ciliary body

Figure 1.1 Classification of uveitis by anatomy.

Just as inflammation can spread from one part of the uveal tract to another it can also spread inwardly and outwardly. To complicate things further the term 'posterior uveitis' is imprecisely and confusingly used to describe inflammation anywhere in the back of the eye and can occur with or without involvement of the choroid. For example, inflammation primarily involving the retina, retinitis, can occur either in isolation, without involvement of the choroid, or secondarily to inflammation in the choroid. Similarly, primary inflammation of the choroid can spread to involve the retina secondarily to cause a retinitis. The same is true for posterior spread to involve the outer coat, the sclera. Endophthalmitis is a condition where the entirety of the inside of the eye is inflamed such that the layer most affected cannot be discerned. In this condition the outermost coat, the sclera, is not yet heavily involved. Panophthalmitis is where the inside of the eye and all three coats are inflamed. Although strictly speaking the uveal tract is one distinct layer of the eye, the term 'uveitis' rather confusingly is often applied to any intraocular inflammation, in much the same way as 'America' can be a term applied to either the country or the continent.

Anterior uveitis, also called iritis as this is the portion of the uveal tract involved, is a very common condition to present to eye casualty. Again we state that the first thing one must do to determine what type of uveitis is present is to determine what anatomical locations are involved and where the primary source of the inflammation is located. This is highlighted as the most common error made that leads to uveitis specialists being called as expert witnesses in medicolegal cases where a posterior uveitis with mild anterior component is seen in eye casualty and treated with topical drops alone. This is almost always due to the casualty officer not dilating the pupil and looking at the fundus, and in turn this is almost always due to time pressure in accident and emergency resulting in corners being cut. If determining the primary source of the inflammation is paramount in working through diagnosis and treatment, this is impossible to do without actually looking at all the sites.

Tip: **Always dilate patients presenting with anterior uveitis and examine the entire eye for inflammation. Always examine both eyes.**

Table 1.1 Classification of uveitis by course of the disease

Time	≤3 months	>3 months
Duration	Limited	Persistent
Separation between episodes – the time between episodes of inflammation when the eye was quiet and the patient was on no treatment	Chronic	Recurrent

CLASSIFICATION BY SEVERITY AND COURSE OF THE DISEASE

The Standardisation of Uveitis Nomenclature (SUN) working group has established specific criteria for determining the severity of flare and cells in the anterior chamber and degree of vitritis in the posterior segment. These will be dealt with in their respective chapters. The course of the disease begins with the **onset** itself and knowing if this was sudden or insidious is important as it can help differentiate between conditions. If the episode lasts less than or equal to 3 months the **duration** is said to be limited and if greater than 3 months persistent. If there are multiple inflammatory episodes separated by more than or equal to 3 months without treatment the condition is said to be recurrent, but if the gap between episodes is less than 3 months it is called chronic (see Table 1.1).

CLASSIFICATION BY CAUSE OF THE DISEASE

The purpose of classifying uveitis when first seeing a patient is to determine its cause. There are legion causes of uveitis which we will discuss as we get to them, but essentially these can be broken down into three categories: infectious, inflammatory and neoplasia mimicking inflammation. The term 'masquerade syndrome' is sometimes used to describe the latter as it presents in a number of ways although there are certain features that are constant and which the initiated can look out for. Clearly the treatment for all three is very different but until it is known for certain which of the three main causes is to blame some basic principles will help guide initial treatment. A patient history is very important here as well and several sensitive questions will need to be asked, although it is not uncommon for a patient with a sexually transmitted element to their eye condition to categorically deny certain facts until presented with their test results. Inflammatory eye disease is one of those strange sub-specialties in which the signs you see and symptoms the patient experiences guide the physician into asking very focused questions that develop the clinical encounter.

NEXT STEPS

Once the patient with uveitis has had their condition classified then long lists of differential diagnoses suddenly become manageable. This book is structured so the reader can now jump to the chapter in question where the logical process of arriving at a diagnosis and appropriate treatment plan can be discussed. Investigations, both clinical and ancillary, are a minefield and before going ahead and ticking every box on the blood form you're about to hand the patient it is well worth reading the next chapter.

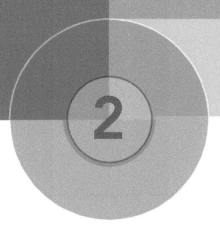

Differentiating between different diagnoses: Clinical and ancillary testing

2

The list of different systemic and local conditions associated with inflammatory eye disease is legion. If an ophthalmologist thinks about the entire list every time they approach a patient then they are likely to get lost very early on and order a battery of tests, which are then likely to cause further diagnostic confusion. The saying 'less is more' is nowhere more relevant than it is here, and the key to a good choice of tests to conduct is an efficient history and a logical approach.

APPROACHING A UVEITIC PATIENT

The first thing to do, as mentioned in Chapter 1, is to classify the uveitis and to determine if it is unilateral or bilateral. If a condition is bilateral then a systemic association is more likely. Depending on how the uveitis is classified, specific things can then be asked, if not already volunteered in the general medical history. Do not ask all patients regardless of classification a question about every single known systemic association. For example, asking a patient with a simple unilateral anterior uveitis whether they have had mouth ulcers is not only pointless, it is dangerous as well. If they say yes how does that help? Does it make a diagnosis of Behçet more likely if they have? The simple answer is no. The patient is worried, and the doctor is confused. Table 2.1 will help direct questions to specific areas.

The patient may volunteer symptoms, but as a general rule the possibility of systemic associations increases the further back the uveitis is present in the eye. Only ask questions if the answer will determine what tests you do and only do tests if the results will determine what treatment you give. For example a patient who has anterior uveitis and who also has associated ankylosing spondylitis is not really going to benefit from a HLA-B27 blood test treatment wise. The patient might benefit, however, from the knowledge that he or she might have a specific back problem that makes the recurrence of the anterior uveitis more likely and can hence prepare for it. Likewise asking about tuberculosis (TB) exposure if you're not preparing to test for TB will only confuse. Choose your questions carefully. Contrary to what some textbooks say we would not readily suggest examining skin rashes, joints or listening to chests. Ophthalmologists are not traditionally very good at these things, and it is better to take the patient at his or her word and if necessary refer to other specialties for their opinion.

Table 2.1 Tailor questions to your findings

Classification	Question	Rationale/association
Anterior uveitis	Do you have back pain?	Ankylosing spondylitis
	Do you have any bowel problems or skin problems?	Crohn's and ulcerative colitis
		Psoriasis
Intermediate uveitis	Do you have any lung or joint problems?	Sarcoidosis, TB
	Do you have any neurological symptoms?	Multiple sclerosis
Posterior uveitis	We ask everyone this question as sometimes eye inflammation can be related to a sexually transmitted disease. How many people have you had sex with in the past 6 months and were they male, female, or both? Did you have protected or unprotected sex and what kind of intercourse did you have?	Syphilis, HIV and related conditions
	Have you had any exposure to TB?	TB
	Have you had oral or genital ulceration?	Behçet
	More specific questions	See Chapter 5

OPTICAL COHERENCE TOMOGRAPHY

Optical coherence tomography (OCT) scanning is very useful in determining if cystoid macular oedema is present and in assessing its severity. It can track the response to treatment and is a very useful test to perform in clinic. In almost all cases of posterior and intermediate uveitis an OCT scan is useful and can help guide treatment though it should only be rarely needed in patients with anterior uveitis such as those with chronic disease or where the vision is worse than expected.

BLOOD TESTS

The false-positive rates with blood tests done for uveitic purposes are such that if many are ordered then the chance of a distracting, clinically unhelpful result goes from a distinct possibility to a near certainty. Antinuclear antibody (ANA) and antineutrophil cytoplasmic antibody (ANCA) are the worst culprits.

RADIOLOGY

A chest x-ray (CXR) is mandatory if doing blood tests for lung-based conditions, specifically sarcoidosis and TB, as it can make the clinical importance of the blood test result more or less powerful. If there is any doubt about the CXR findings a computed tomography (CT) scan of the thorax is very well placed in giving a detailed result that can significantly assist treatment. A magnetic resonance imaging (MRI) scan is usually performed for two main reasons: (1) If the patient has neurological symptoms and demyelination or the neurological manifestation of an inflammatory disorder is suspected and (2) in largely asymptomatic patients where intra-ocular lymphoma is suspected, to look for intracranial lesions. Other radiological tests, such as x-rays of diseased joints or of the spinal column, should not be performed by ophthalmologists and if such disease is suspected the patient should be referred to the relevant specialty. Ultrasonography of the eye can be undertaken if there is no fundal view afforded due to debris in the vitreous, or to look for posterior scleral thickening or fluid under Tenon's capsule, the 'T-sign', in suspected posterior scleritis.

FLUORESCEIN AND INDOCYANINE GREEN ANGIOGRAPHY

These tests can be useful in patients with posterior uveitis for both diagnostic and treatment purposes. Certain conditions have very distinctive appearances on angiography which can assist diagnosis and hence treatment. In occlusive vascular conditions that may have associated neovascularisation angiography can reveal areas of peripheral ischaemia that can help guide the application of panretinal photocoagulation (PRP) laser. In other conditions angiography can give an indication of the patient's response to treatment; for example a vasculitis with leakage and vessel staining on angiography subsequently treated with immunosuppressive medications may have repeat angiography to assess the response, and management can then be guided with regard to dose or medication alterations.

SKIN TESTS

The only skin test ophthalmologists are ever likely to come across is the Mantoux test for TB and this is best done via the respiratory physicians. Other textbooks mention myriad other skin tests such as the pathergy test, but none of this is useful as these have been long abandoned in the West. A skin biopsy can be considered a test of sorts, and where skin granulomas are present in a suspected case of sarcoidosis a referral to dermatology for a biopsy can give an invaluable tissue diagnosis.

VITREOUS BIOPSY

In cases of suspected intraocular infection a vitreous biopsy, or 'tap', is an important test. Principally the test is done to look for bacteria or viruses and is done in the following manner:

1. Perform the test in a clean room.
2. Place oxybuprocaine drops in the patient's eye, followed by 5% iodine, as per preparation for an intravitreal injection.
3. Apply 10% iodine skin preparation, followed by a sterile drape and speculum.
4. Apply another drop of oxybuprocaine.
5. Advance a 1 mL syringe and orange needle (25 gauge) into the vitreous 4 mm posterior to the limbus and withdraw 0.3 mL of fluid.
6. If this is not possible, 'dry tap', try gently advancing the needle, turning the bevel, or angling the needle slightly posteriorly. Failing this, withdrawing and repeating the procedure with a blue needle (23 gauge) can be considered. If it is still not possible do not persist.
7. Withdraw needle and prepare sample.

It is important to note here that knowing how your local laboratory likes the sample prepared is important to deduce **before** the procedure is undertaken. Some laboratories like the needle removed, the syringe capped and the whole sent to them while others prefer the oph-thalmologist to decant aliquots of fluid into separate syringes before sending as they go to separate departments for culture, virology and polymerase chain reaction (PCR). It is a very common mistake to do the procedure flawlessly and then prepare the sample incorrectly such that only a few of the important tests are performed. By the time the mistake is realised the patient has been on treatment and repeating the procedure is almost always not possible. If the tap is to be undertaken at the same time as an injection of antibiotic it is vital to prepare this beforehand (see Chapter 6). Although it is perfectly natural for the eye to be soft after the procedure excessive softness can lead to other problems as an inflamed eye might be unable to quickly replace the volume due to ciliary body involvement.

AQUEOUS BIOPSY

This is the vitreous biopsy's little brother. It is easier to perform but diagnostically less useful due to the small volume of fluid obtained and the high false-negative rate. The procedure is as follows:

1. The test is performed at the slit lamp.
2. Place oxybuprocaine drops in the patient's eye, followed by 5% iodine, as per preparation for an intravitreal injection.
3. Insert a lid speculum.
4. Position the patient at the slit lamp with or without the support of an assistant and focus on the anterior chamber.
5. Advance a 1 mL syringe with grey needle (27 gauge) into the anterior chamber from just in front of the limbus and parallel to the iris, bevel (open end of needle) towards you.
6. Withdraw the plunger very slowly, watching carefully for anterior chamber collapse and avoid touching any structures. The maximum amount of fluid that can be withdrawn is 0.2 mL.
7. Withdraw needle and prepare sample.

The note above about sample preparation still stands, though it is only usually PCR that can be performed on this sample as it is so small in volume.

ELECTRODIAGNOSTIC TESTS

In the field of uveitis electrodiagnostic tests (EDTs) are almost exclusively restricted to moni-toring patients with birdshot chorioretinopathy (see Chapter 5) where comparison of yearly electroretinograms gives a good indication of whether the patient is immunosuppressed enough.

DECISION-MAKING IN UVEITIC PATIENTS

The principles of managing patients with inflammatory eye disease come first and the diag-nosis commonly comes last. Managing a terrorist attack is somewhat similar the world over and although it is very useful to know the nature of the terrorists and what their demands are these things can usually wait until the attack itself has been brought under control by local law enforcement. Knowing the group they belong to is mostly useful in knowing how to avoid further attacks. Similarly, if we get bogged down trying to work out the exact diagnosis before commencing treatment patients will suffer irreversible vision loss as the inflammatory process damages the eye. There are a few specific patterns to be aware of and these will be discussed in the next few chapters. Keep blood tests to a minimum and always remember, 'less is more'.

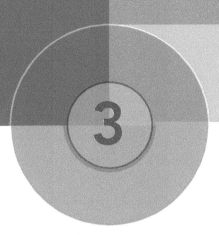

Anterior uveitis

3

Anterior uveitis makes up the vast majority of uveitis cases seen in eye casualty. The proportion varies between 60% and 90% with the smallest units possessing the greatest percentages of anterior uveitis making up the uveitis case mix, as they are the least likely to be referred on to tertiary centres. It is the first form of uveitis the ophthalmologist in training comes across and the easiest to treat. Due to this relative ease of diagnosis and treatment it is sadly not uncommon for corners to be cut and mistakes to be made. If time is taken to properly classify the disease then these pitfalls can be avoided. Table 3.1 can be used as an aide-memoir.

The most common mistake made in treating anterior uveitis is when the patient does not have anterior uveitis, but anterior signs from a posterior uveitis. This is why every patient presenting with uveitis **must** have their fundus and posterior segment checked for inflammation. If there are signs of inflammation in the fundus, vasculitis or snowballs present the patient does not have anterior uveitis. The only posterior feature that anterior uveitis is allowed to have is cystoid macular oedema (CMO), which can occur if the inflammation is severe and long lasting. It must be remembered however that spillover from severe anterior uveitis can also cause cells to appear in the anterior vitreous, though in much lower concentrations.

This may be the first attack or it may be the latest in a long line of attacks. If the latter then either the same eye is always involved or the attacks can alternate. If it is always the same eye that is involved it is essential to look for signs of a viral aetiology such as iris defects or corneal involvement that may signify a herpetic element. Attacks that alternate where one eye is involved then the other is typical of HLA-B27 disease. Approximately 50% of patients presenting with acute anterior uveitis (AAU) are HLA-B27 positive and 50% are negative, while around 8% of the Caucasian general population is positive. If a patient is HLA-B27 positive the attacks are said to be more frequent and more severe although as the treatment is much the same knowing this fact is of dubious importance. The patient might however be reassured to know that there is a cause for the recurrent attacks of uveitis, even if the treatment is the same, and knowledge of HLA-B27 positivity might avoid further less useful investigations down the line. If the disease is bilateral at the same time then a systemic condition such as sarcoidosis is more likely and a careful history and examination of the posterior segment should be conducted to make doubly sure that it is purely an anterior uveitis that one is dealing with. On second glance it is not too uncommon to find a snowball or two in the inferior vitreous in bilateral cases which automatically turns the condition into an intermediate uveitis, which makes Chapter 4 the chapter for you.

Attacks of anterior uveitis are typically limited and recurrent as opposed to persistent (lasts longer than 3 months) and chronic (treatment-free gap between episodes is less than 3 months).

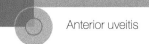

Table 3.1 Classification of anterior uveitis

Anatomical location	Is it definitely anterior uveitis?
Laterality	Unilateral, bilateral, alternating?
Duration	Limited or persistent?
Course	Chronic or recurrent?
Severity	See Tables 3.3 and 3.4

If this is not the case, and especially if it is always one eye involved, look carefully for signs of a herpetic cause.

DIAGNOSIS

The diagnosis is a clinical one. The features to look out for in the history are classically **photophobia, mild blur** and **pain**. The important signs are **ciliary injection**, where the redness is worse immediately surrounding the limbus as this is the location of the ciliary body; **keratic precipitates** (KPs), which are inflammatory debris that appear in spots on the corneal endothelium; and anterior chamber **cells, flare** and **hypopyon**. KPs are sometimes termed 'granulomatous' or 'non-granulomatous' with the granulomatous variety said to be bigger, more greasy looking and more likely to be associated with sarcoidosis, tuberculosis and leprosy. In reality this distinction is unhelpful and it is vanishingly rare for any of these three conditions to be diagnosed based on the type of KPs a person has during an otherwise straightforward attack of anterior uveitis. An important variant of keratic precipitates, and possibly the only clinically relevant variant, are the 'stellate' KPs that are associated with Fuchs heterochromic iridocyclitis. Stellate is Latin for 'star' as the appearances of the KPs on the corneal endothelium resemble the night sky with an even distribution of small dots all over the cornea as if looking up at the night sky. The standard pattern is for the KPs to be located more inferiorly and to be bigger. Figure 3.1 illustrates the difference between normally distributed KPs and stellate KPs.

Cells are leucocytes that can be seen idling in and out of a highly magnified and brightly illuminated slice of aqueous humour much like dust particles passing in and out of a bright beam of sunlight in an old room. Flare implies a breakdown of the blood-aqueous barrier as protein and fibrin that have leaked into the aqueous have a blurring effect on what we see in and what the patient sees out. A hypopyon is an inferior collection of inflammatory material at the bottom of the anterior chamber which is a sign of severity. It is traditionally measured by vertical height at the slit lamp.

The iris is an important structure to examine in detail and Table 3.2 gives an overview of what to look for and the relevance of various signs. Iris nodules may be located in the body of the iris or at the pupil margin. Those in the middle away from the pupil margin are termed 'Busacca nodules' and those at the edge of the pupil are termed 'Koeppe nodules', which can be remembered by thinking that people who cannot Koeppe are usually on the edge.

All uveitis patients should have their intraocular pressures measured due to the association of glaucoma with intraocular inflammation. Uveitis can cause the pressure to rise through inflammatory debris blocking the trabecular meshwork, inflammation of the trabecular meshwork itself, a 'zipping shut' of the meshwork and blocking of the angle due to ongoing inflammation and pupillary block due to 360° posterior synechiae. This latter condition is termed 'iris bombe' due to a similarity between the appearance of the billowed out iris and the popular dessert. Additionally a steroid response to the treatments that we start may cause a rise in pressure.

Tip: Always measure the intraocular pressure of uveitis patients at each visit.

(a)

(b)

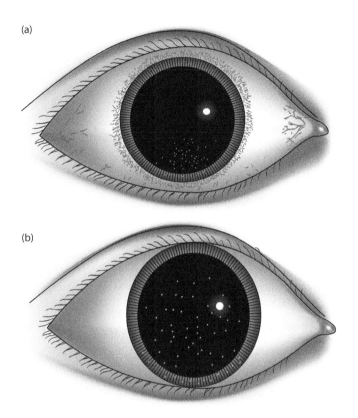

Figure 3.1 (a) Keratic precipitate distribution in AAU and (b) stellate keratic precipitates in Fuchs heterochromic iridocyclitis.

Table 3.2 Iris pathology in acute anterior uveitis

Iris sign	Relevance
Sectoral iris atrophy	Varicella zoster virus (VZV)
Patchy iris atrophy	Herpes simplex virus (HSV)
Iris nodules	Sarcoidosis, TB
Posterior synechiae	Extremely unlikely to be Fuchs heterochromic iridocyclitis
Heterochromia	Likely to be Fuchs heterochromic iridocyclitis

SEVERITY

Once you're certain that the patient in front of you has anterior uveitis it is important to then grade the severity. This is so the response to treatment can be measured and for proper communication between different physicians who may see the patient at different visits. The Standardisation of Uveitis Nomenclature (SUN) working group developed specific guidelines so that this can be achieved and to stop the non-specific 'mild, moderate and severe' that is of no use in modern ophthalmology. The severity is mainly measured through two indicators, cells and flare. Cells are actual observed leucocytes in the anterior chamber, a testament to the magnification ability of the slit lamp. They are best observed by using high magnification

Table 3.3 Anterior chamber cell grading according to the SUN classification

Number of cells observed in 1 mm by 1 mm beam	Cell grading
0	–
1–5	+/–
6–15	+
16–25	++
26–50	+++
>50	++++

and high luminance and then shining a beam of 1 mm by 1 mm light at a slight angle, usually around 30° from the axis of the slit lamp, into the eye and focusing anterior to the pupillary plane such that no iris or other structure is visible, only aqueous. Aqueous is of course invisible but any cells that may be present drift in and out of the beam of light in a convection current. The severity of the inflammation measured by the number of cells you can count in the 1 mm by 1 mm beam of light has been standardised by the SUN working group as summarised in Table 3.3. Note that the cells may be clear or pigmented, with clear cells representing fresh inflammation and pigmented cells representing old inflammation, the presence of which is regarded as more of a red herring to trap the uninitiated into thinking active inflammation is present when there is not rather than being significant in themselves.

In practice, despite this official classification, people generally do not laboriously count the cells as this is difficult because the cells are constantly moving. They pretend they do to obey the SUN criteria so how much of an advancement this is in reality is difficult to ascertain. The second criterion in the measurement of severity is flare. Flare is a measure of the protein content of the aqueous which itself is a measure of the permeability of the blood retina/aqueous barrier which again is a measure of the level of inflammation present. If there is much inflammation there is much protein leakage and thus increased blur when looking at the iris as the protein affects the turbidity of the fluid. If the breakdown in the blood-aqueous barrier is sufficiently serious then fibrin can congeal the protein into a pale translucent blob that sits in the anterior chamber and often obscures the pupil. This automatically promotes the flare into a grade 4 flare, the most advanced kind. Flare is graded as per Table 3.4.

When measuring the severity of anterior uveitis the main two measures used are therefore cells and flare. Secondary measures include vertical height of hypopyon (if present) and vertical height of the fibrin clot (if present). Degree of pain, photophobia, injection, keratic precipitates and all else are not used for grading severity or response to treatment although they are

Table 3.4 Anterior chamber flare grading according to the SUN classification

Degree of blur looking at the iris	Flare grading
None	–
Hardly any	+
Definite blur but iris details still clear	++
Obvious blur with iris details hazy	+++
Fibrinous flare/plastic aqueous	++++

commonly noted. As with pigmented cells indicating old inactive uveitis, pigmented keratic precipitates indicate previous rather than current inflammation.

INVESTIGATIONS

This is controversial, and uveitis specialists differ quite significantly on how this is approached. Some investigate all cases of anterior uveitis, others none. Others abide by an 'investigate on the third attack' or 'only if it is bilateral' rule. There must always be reasons for the choices we make and before deciding there are a few important questions to ask:

1. Is it *anterior* uveitis for sure? This point has been laboured but it is very important. If it is anterior uveitis then the need for investigation diminishes dramatically.
2. Are there any systemic symptoms? If so then will doing a test make an investigation for a particular condition matter? For example if there is absolutely no systemic complaint will a borderline or even raised angiotensin-converting enzyme (ACE) change anything in your management or even mean anything? The answer is no.
3. If there are systemic symptoms such as back pain, Crohn's disease or psoriasis indicative of HLA-B27 disease should this be tested for? Again, if it does not change what you do there is no point in doing this test. Unless the back pain was such that a positive result might mean referral to a rheumatologist for ankylosing spondylitis then yes, but if not, no.
4. If it is a 'granulomatous' anterior uveitis should this be investigated? Nodules in the iris or thick greasy KPs might be indicative of sarcoidosis, tuberculosis (TB) or leprosy but again point 2 still stands. If there is no systemic symptom what will you then do with borderline or even positive results?
5. Could the person have a systemic symptom they are unwilling to divulge? Could the uveitis be a manifestation of a sexually transmitted infection such as syphilis? This might need some further digging. Have a low threshold for asking a sexual history and if positive, or even if not sufficiently negative, investigate accordingly.

Tip: **Only investigate if your results will alter management.**

SPECIFIC ANTERIOR UVEITIS ENTITIES THAT DO NOT REQUIRE INVESTIGATION

Sometimes anterior uveitis is part of a local syndrome where the diagnosis is clinical. There are three main diagnoses here: Fuchs heterochromic iridocyclitis, also called Fuchs uveitis syndrome, Posner-Schlossman syndrome and herpetic uveitis, and an anterior segment ischaemia syndrome. There are some very simple questions that can be asked that can help you differentiate between these three classes of disease:

1. Are the irises different colours? If so think of Fuchs heterochromic iridocyclitis. Note here however that although heterochromia is indeed incorporated into the very name of this condition this sign itself is considered increasingly unreliable in the uveitis community.
2. Is the intraocular pressure unusually high? If so think of Posner-Schlossman syndrome.
3. Is there any other ocular pathology present such as severe diabetic retinopathy, vein occlusion, previous muscle surgery or ocular ischaemic syndrome? If so consider that the uveitis is secondary to this.

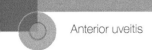
FUCHS

Fuchs is a peculiar condition that is very important to recognise. Prompt diagnosis can save the patient from unnecessary investigations, can spare the patient harmful treatment in the form of steroids and can also allow the clinician to make a confident prognosis. It is usually unilateral but can be bilateral in up to 10% of cases. There are key features present that help the ophthalmologist make the correct identification: the inflammation is chronic and low grade; this means that they never present to the emergency department with a red eye, pain or photophobia. The patients usually present via the optometrist who may notice 'inflammation' incorrectly diagnosed as anterior uveitis, a cataract or raised intraocular pressure. Sometimes these signs are discovered incidentally during an eye exam at the hospital when the patient presents with an unrelated condition. The key signs are a white eye with chronic anterior chamber activity in the absence of posterior synechiae. Other key signs are stellate keratic precipitates and iris atrophy.

If Fuchs is suspected look for iris stromal atrophy and compare especially with the fellow unaffected eye. The iris takes on a rather 'moth-eaten' appearance and iris nodules may be seen in the stroma. It is this atrophy that causes iris heterochromia, hence the name, but as this is an unreliable finding it should not be over-relied upon. Anterior vitreous cells are common but very occasionally the vitritis can be very dense. This can mislead the clinician and has in some cases caused a missed diagnosis, which resulted in the patient being inappropriately treated with systemic steroids or even immunosuppression. By definition however despite the apparent severity of the vitreitis cystoid macular oedema is never present. A final curious finding in Fuchs is that fluorescein angiography will often show optic disc uptake of fluorescein dye, called a disc flush when compared to the contralateral unaffected eye. For this reason performing a fluorescein angiogram can be a useful additional test in cases of doubt.

Even though happily patients with Fuchs do not require treatment for the cells present in the anterior chamber they must still be followed up as development of glaucoma is a very real risk and cataract surgery will be needed at some stage. About a quarter of patients have raised intraocular pressure at the time of their Fuchs diagnosis. Thereafter the subsequent incidence of new glaucoma during follow up is quite low. It is thought to be caused by the rubella virus in some way but nobody really knows.

POSNER-SCHLOSSMAN SYNDROME

Posner-Schlossman syndrome is characterised by episodes of very high intraocular pressure in one eye in, typically, a young male patient which recur every so often with very little in the way of inflammation. The giveaway sign is meant to be very small, sparse KPs. You can be a hero when asked about an apparent episode of angle closure where the angle is open and you announce the correct diagnosis after detecting the KPs. Treatment is with corticosteroid drops, as below, and anti-glaucoma medication. A cycloplegic is not needed as, like Fuchs, the inflammation almost never reaches a level severe enough to cause posterior synechiae formation. It is thought that cytomegalovirus (CMV) is the causative agent in some of these patients. This occurs in otherwise healthy, immunocompetent subjects, usually males. It appears to be much more prevalent in Asia, for example Singapore, Japan and Korea, although the authors have seen cases in the UK. CMV anterior uveitis causes a Possner-Schlossman phenotype, characterised by recurrent attacks of hypertensive uveitis, with sparse KPs, and minimal if any posterior synechiae formation. It tends to be resistant to topical steroids and this feature should alert the clinician to suspect CMV infection. The virus can sometimes be identified on an AC tap when the disease is active. If recognised early, patients can do well if treated with topical Ganciclovir gel 0.15%, applied initially every 2 hours for 2 weeks, then tapered to tds maintenance. Treatment must be prolonged over many months and relapses are common.

Likewise recurrent unilateral anterior uveitis may be associated with **herpes simplex virus** (HSV) or **varicella zoster virus** (VZV), the clue being patchy iris atrophy in the former and sectoral atrophy in the latter. The main clue though, like the diagnoses above, is the unilaterality of the inflammation. Knowing which virus is the cause is unimportant as the treatment is the same; topical steroids as detailed below and an oral antiviral usually for 2 weeks, either in the form of acyclovir 800 mg five times a day or valaciclovir 1 g three times a day (tds). Should the eye flare up more than twice a year prophylaxis with acyclovir 400 mg twice daily (bd) can be employed. According to the herpetic eye disease study prophylaxis can reduce the frequency of recurrences by up to 50% while used. A topical antiviral, usually in the form of acyclovir ointment, is entirely useless unless by some coincidence the cornea is also involved.

If there is persistent anterior uveitis in an eye with a known ocular pathology always consider a link between the two. **Ischaemic** conditions in particular can cause a breakdown in the blood-aqueous barrier, and there is a very long list of conditions that cause ischaemia. Essentially if the patient has a recurrent unilateral anterior uveitis and a concurrent ischaemic syndrome then consider long-term prophylactic topical steroid therapy and a cycloplegic, classically dexamethasone 0.1% (Maxidex) bd and atropine 1% once daily (od).

WHY TREAT ANTERIOR UVEITIS?

Before doing anything, particularly embarking on a course of therapy with potential side effects, it is essential to know why it is being done. The aim of treatment is to eliminate the inflammation to treat pain and photophobia in the short term and prevent glaucoma, cataract and posterior synechiae formation in the medium to long term. Patients should be aware of the risks of not treating the disease as it is very common, particularly in young people, for ongoing inflammation to fox the ophthalmologist when all along the drops are being administered rarely if at all.

TREATMENT

Treating anterior uveitis has two aspects: treating the actual uveitis and preventing complications from the uveitis. This second category includes preventing posterior synechiae formation by giving cyclopentolate 1% to dilate the pupil for the active duration of the inflammation and treating any high intraocular pressure that might occur with a drop such as timolol 0.5% bd. In simple cases of anterior uveitis without extensive posterior synechiae formation, Table 3.5 demonstrates a standard regime. Dexamethasone 0.1% drops (Maxidex) or prednisolone acetate 1% (Pred Forte) are interchangeable. Occasionally a steroid ointment is given before bed but if the patient follows the regime this is not needed.

If the anterior uveitis recurs or indeed never properly settled then the regime can be repeated with each step lasting 2 weeks rather than 1 week. If the patient has significant posterior synechiae that do not break with dilation on the initial visit then the usual option is to wait a week and review, then to see if a week of dilating drops has done the trick. If this is not the case then injecting 0.5 mL of **subconjunctival mydricaine**, a mixture of atropine, adrenaline and

Table 3.5 Treatment regime for simple acute anterior uveitis

Drop frequency	Duration
Dexamethasone (Maxidex) hourly	1 week
Cyclopentolate 1% tds	1 week then stop
Dexamethasone (Maxidex) every 2 hours	1 week
Qds	1 week
Tds	1 week
Bd	1 week
Od	1 week

procaine, can help break the synechiae. This is done in the following manner, either at the slit lamp or lying down (Figure 3.2):

1. Numb the eye with a few drops of oxybuprocaine followed by 5% iodine into the palpebral fissure.
2. Insert a lid speculum.
3. Ask the patient to look in the most convenient direction and with toothed forceps in one hand and the 1 mL syringe containing 0.5 mL of mydricaine in the other with short orange needle attached grasp the conjunctiva with the forceps and inject with bevel towards you (open end of needle) the whole amount under the conjunctiva.
4. The closer to the limbus this is done the better though paradoxically due to the anatomy this is in fact easiest the further away from the limbus the injection takes place. Try and inject the whole 0.5 mL if you can (Figure 3.2).

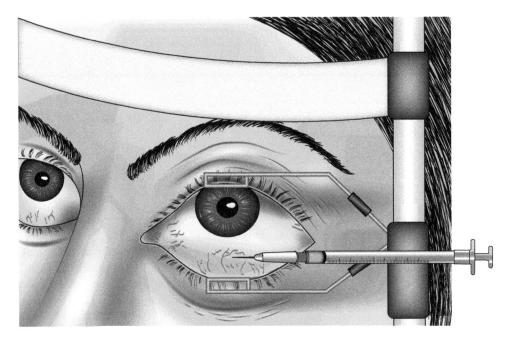

Figure 3.2 Subconjunctival injection of mydricaine at the slit lamp.

Similarly, subconjunctival injection of **Betnesol** (betamethasone sodium phosphate 0.1%) may help if the inflammation does not settle after a week or two, is worsening or compliance is an issue. This is performed in the same manner as above except 1 mL (4 mg) is injected.

FOLLOW-UP

For first attacks of anterior uveitis it is prudent to follow the patient up in a week or two following the initiation of therapy to check improvement, measure intraocular pressure and examine again the posterior segment for activity. If all is well then one final follow-up 6–8 weeks later to ensure the eye is quiet off all medication is good practice, after which the patient can be discharged. If the condition is worsening always check compliance, particularly in young people and in men and in young men in particular. In a worsening situation on hourly drops a subconjunctival steroid injection as detailed above or commencement of half hourly drops may be needed. It is very unusual to require oral steroids in a simple anterior uveitis but at each visit the fundus must be examined to ensure the situation is still quiet in the posterior segment.

For a second attack of anterior uveitis, if the first was treated without issue, then a single follow-up in 6 weeks should be sufficient with the proviso that the patient contacts the department in the event of any problem. From the third attack onwards if there have been no pressure issues or steroid response then the patient can be discharged at the first visit if they can be relied upon to contact eye casualty in the event of a problem.

CHRONIC ANTERIOR UVEITIS

Sometimes anterior uveitis will flare up again within 3 months if the drops are stopped or even when the drops are reduced to the once a day stage. Patients will even say things like 'I am fine until I get down to once a day then I have to go back up again.' The mistake that ophthalmologists commonly make is to persist in trying to stop the drops. Once it is clear that the patient has chronic uveitis, a conclusion reached after stopping the drops has been attempted at least three times with increasingly gentle tapering regimes, then a form of long-term therapy can be considered. The main two ocular risks of long-term topical steroid therapy, cataracts and glaucoma will always need to be borne in mind and the patient monitored for these things at 3- to 4-month intervals for the entire duration of treatment.

A course of long-term topical steroid therapy for anterior uveitis will be dependent on the drop frequency at which the patient flared up. Table 3.6 outlines suggested long-term therapy regimens.

Should pressure become an issue or cataracts start to develop alternatives to Maxidex can be employed in the form of a weaker steroid such as fluorometholone (FML) or a non-steroidal

Table 3.6 Long-term therapy regimens for chronic anterior uveitis

Drop frequency at which flare-up occurred	Drop frequency for long-term therapy
Bd Maxidex	Tds Maxidex
Od Maxidex	Bd Maxidex
Alternate day Maxidex	Od Maxidex
After cessation	Alternate day Maxidex

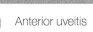
such as nepafenac (Nevanac) or ketorolac (Acular). These are weaker and as such have fewer side effects as well and may be used instead of topical steroid to prevent flare-ups. Regimes are usually tds, bd or od and the benefit of the non-steroidal is that these patients can be followed up less frequently in clinic. It might be useful to consider a drop of non-steroidal to be approximately equal to a half or third of the potency of Maxidex at controlling inflammation.

After 6 months of being quiet it might then be possible to again try to wean the patient off the drop but should this result in a flare-up the drops can be continued indefinitely, though further attempts at weaning at least once every 2 years is recommended.

CONSIDERATIONS IN CHILDREN

Although uveitis is a disease of younger patients the peak onset is in early adulthood and early middle age as opposed to childhood. If the patient in front of you is less than 16 years of age, or if they are a little older but the condition started before the patient was 16, consider juvenile idiopathic arthritis (JIA). In fact it can be argued that the importance of this condition cannot be overestimated in this age group and perhaps a better way of thinking about it is to assume that anterior uveitis in this age group is JIA until proven otherwise. The key with this condition is that patients have arthritis affecting a few joints and the uveitis is entirely asymptomatic with no pain at all. The uveitis is typically chronic anterior uveitis and is usually bilateral, although it can be asymmetrical. All the usual sequelae of chronic untreated inflammation occur – cataract, glaucoma, posterior synechiae and even band keratopathy – but the only symptoms will be blurred vision and sometimes floaters. Posterior segment signs of inflammation are usually absent, but in severe cases sometimes inflammatory cells can spillover into the anterior vitreous and cystoids macular oedema can develop. The lack of symptoms means that the disease may have caused a lot of damage by the time it presents to an ophthalmologist and for this reason patients are screened by us to look for inflammation. Note that the eye may appear quite inflamed when looking for cells and flare, though there will be no ciliary injection and the eye will look white. There will be no need to diagnose the condition, as this will have been done by the rheumatologists or paediatricians and will become immediately obvious in the history.

Around 30% of JIA patients overall can suffer from uveitis but the figure is higher if:

1. Less than four joints are affected, called oligoarticular disease
2. ANA status is positive

The screening schedule is every 2 months from the onset of the arthritis then every 4 months until the child is 12 years old, and if the child is older than 12 then for a year. Should the eye become inflamed then the treatment is the same as with an adult initially but can become complex with secondary glaucoma and cataract becoming big problems. Immunosuppression may be needed, with methotrexate being an option in children. In recalcitrant cases biologics are also used, but really from this point onwards the child should be in the care of a paediatric uveitis specialist and our duty as non-specialists is to start treatment and refer in a timely manner.

CONSIDERATIONS IN CATARACT SURGERY

Patients with recurrent anterior uveitis are more likely to develop cataract and when they undergo cataract surgery they are more likely to develop a flare-up of anterior uveitis as a result of the surgery. Indeed patients with no history of uveitis would almost universally develop inflammation were it not for post-operative steroid drops. In patients with known previous attacks of anterior uveitis it is prudent to wait 3 months after an attack has ended before undergoing cataract surgery with the timer resetting if an attack should happen in the meantime. Covering a patient with a week of four times a day dexamethasone 0.1% (Maxidex) in the run-up to the operation and treating the patient as per the regime in Table 3.5 post-operatively would reduce the chance of a large flare-up of uveitis induced by the operation. Topical non-steroidal anti-inflammatory drops such as ketorolac (Acular) four times a day for 6 weeks also have a role to play in the run-up to the operation as well as in the post-operative period.

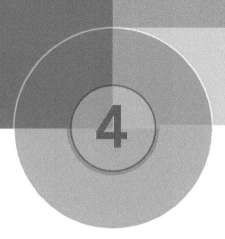

Intermediate uveitis

Intermediate uveitis is said to be present when the primary focus for the inflammation is in the ciliary body and anterior vitreous. The old name for intermediate uveitis, 'peripheral uveitis', is perhaps useful as well as it characterises the condition as a particular form of posterior uveitis in which the signs are only to be seen very peripherally in the posterior segment. As with anything that is not specifically one thing or another there is some confusion surrounding this condition with an alternative name 'pars planitis', which in fact describes a particular subset of patients within this group, sometimes being used interchangeably to describe any patient with intermediate uveitis. Probably the simplest definition of intermediate uveitis is inflammation in which the anterior vitreous is more involved than the anterior chamber and in which there may be very peripheral retinal signs present. It accounts for up to 15% of all cases of uveitis.

All cases of anterior uveitis should be dilated and the entire posterior segment, including the anterior vitreous and posterior retina, examined carefully for signs. Approximately 80% of cases are bilateral as well so if signs are seen in one eye the other should be carefully re-examined to look for even the smallest snowball or scantiest anterior vitreous cells present, should none have been found the first time. Classically intermediate uveitis as opposed to anterior uveitis has a greater tendency to be chronic though there is a paradoxically lower incidence of secondary glaucoma.

From the perspective of the ophthalmologist about to examine a patient with supposed anterior uveitis in eye casualty there are a few clues that can help in the history to guide you.

HISTORY

While anterior uveitis presents with predictable photophobia, blur and pain which usually prompt the patient to seek help shortly after the condition starts, intermediate uveitis is more likely to present with gradual blurriness and increasing floaters. Pain may be a feature but rarely if ever reaches the same level as it does in anterior uveitis. The reason for this is that in anterior uveitis the iris is the primary source of the inflammation and shining a light in the eye, which causes the iris to constrict, is painful. With intermediate uveitis the primary source of the inflammation is the ciliary body rather than the iris, so photophobia is much less of a problem, much like moving a broken leg is painful if the bone inside is broken but moving the leg when the broken bone is in the arm is usually not so painful. Likewise using a mydriatic such as cyclopentolate helps with the pain of anterior uveitis by preventing movement as a splint helps

Table 4.1 Differences in history between anterior and intermediate uveitis

Anterior uveitis	Intermediate uveitis
Photophobia	Blurred vision
Pain	Floaters
Blurred vision	Asymptomatic

a broken leg by keeping it in one position. There is hence usually no need for mydriatics if the inflammation is in the ciliary body.

Usually the patient seeks help after their optometrist notes anterior chamber cells during a routine examination and sends the patient in as an anterior uveitis, or the patient notices increasing floaters and blurriness and seeks help themselves. This important distinction in history should alert the ophthalmologist to the possibility of an intermediate uveitis right from the outset. Table 4.1 summarises the important differences in history between anterior and intermediate uveitis.

Interestingly, while in a child anterior uveitis commonly presents with the symptoms of intermediate uveitis in an adult, intermediate uveitis itself can present with pain, photophobia and redness much like an anterior uveitis in an adult. Table 4.1 can therefore be inverted in a child, symptom wise, though this is not always the case and a thorough examination is sacrosanct.

EXAMINATION

Intermediate uveitis by definition involves inflammation of the vitreous, with the inflammation worse in the anterior vitreous. If there is no inflammation of the vitreous to be found then the patient does not have this condition.

The first and most important thing to do when approaching a patient with uveitis is to classify this condition, and we start at the front of the eye and work our way back. It is common to see some anterior signs in the form of a mild anterior uveitis with cells and flare, but usually not anything much more exciting than this. Next, it is important to examine the anterior vitreous and this is best done at the slit lamp where the beam of light is shone through the pupil directly in line with the viewing angle to create a retroillumination effect. This is a field of red filling the dilated pupil which shows up anything that may be floating in between the retina and lens. If the focus is pushed back from the anterior chamber through the lens to the anterior vitreous itself any debris or cells will then become very apparent. If the field of red, the red reflex, remains an unadulterated red with no object blocking your view then either there is no inflammation present or it is very low grade inflammation that you will find when looking peripherally. If intermediate uveitis is present you will see small round **cells** stuck in the anterior vitreous and sheets of opaque material, much like a cobweb, stretching in wavy bands of any possible orientation across your view. Angling the slit lamp beam slightly off centre will allow you to see these signs in greater detail. The slit lamp view of these **vitreous bands** is shown in Figure 4.1.

Now these phenomena may be present in anterior uveitis as well, but the key is to work out which is worse, the anterior or intermediate signs, as well as taking the history into account. If the anterior uveitis is severe then it is common to see cells and debris in the anterior vitreous though these would be fairly mild. If the cells and **debris** in the vitreous are substantial but the anterior chamber only has a few cells then anterior uveitis is not the problem.

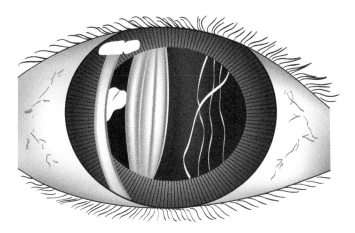

Figure 4.1 Intermediate uveitis from the slit lamp, focussed on the anterior vitreous.

After the anterior vitreous is examined it is then time to examine the fundus, which is where the diagnosis of intermediate uveitis will really be confirmed. It is a combination of what is unaffected as well as what is affected and the old term 'peripheral uveitis' should be remembered here as it nicely illustrates that the signs are, well, peripheral. If there are posterior signs present in the fundus, other than cystoid macular oedema, this is not a case of intermediate uveitis. The hallmark sign of intermediate uveitis is the presence of **snowballs**. These are yellowish condensations of inflammatory material, including macrophages and lymphocytes, that accumulate in the vitreous classically above and not in contact with the inferior retina. They cast a shadow on the retina itself and if located sufficiently far away from it can be seen to move independently when the eye turns. Much as the term 'snowball' implies, the condensations are round and slightly fluffy at the edges. It is also important to remember that the disease is bilateral in 80% of cases but can be very asymmetrical so if snowballs are found in one eye having previously examined the other, going back to re-examine the inferior fundus can often yield a snowball or two that was previously overlooked.

If the disease worsens then a **snowbank** may form, which is actually a collection of exudates forming at the extreme periphery, the level of the ora serrata, which while usually worse inferiorly in extreme cases may be present around the entire circumference of the eye. This is an accumulation of collapsed collagen from degraded vitreous and inflammatory material which sits on the surface of the retina itself and does not float above it as a snowball does. The fact that both entities have 'snow' in the name can and does confuse people into thinking that a snowbank is simply really bad snowballs, but this is not the case. The location of a snowbank is so peripheral that indirect ophthalmoscopy with indentation may be the only way one is found, unless it is particularly bad. It is worth looking for one however if your index of suspicion is high as finding a snowbank is absolute confirmation that you are dealing with an intermediate uveitis. Using a three mirror is easier although less likely to reveal a snowbank than indirect ophthalmoscopy with indentation. Figure 4.2 illustrates how snowballs and snowbanks appear to the ophthalmologist.

While the vessels at the posterior pole should be entirely normal if intermediate as opposed to posterior uveitis is present, there may be signs of **peripheral retinal vasculitis**. This is almost always of peripheral veins, although arterioles may rarely be involved. **Sheathing** of these venules is said to take place, which is a term readily recognised but rarely understood by the ophthalmologist in training. A sheath is a glistening thin-walled covering and the most commonly thought

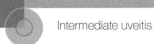
(a)   (b)

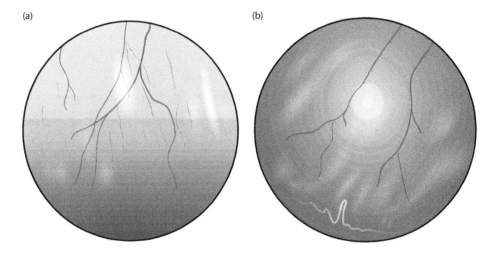

Figure 4.2 (a) Snowballs and (b) snowbank.

of sheath is the simple condom. Imagine a thin covering of inflammatory cells and materials surrounding the venule, more readily seen on either side than on top of the vessel itself, which appears as thin lines either side of but not separated from the vessel but in this condition is only found in the most peripheral vessels. Imagine the vessel with a condom on. Figure 4.3 illustrates peripheral sheathing. As the sheath is constructed of inflammatory cells that have escaped from

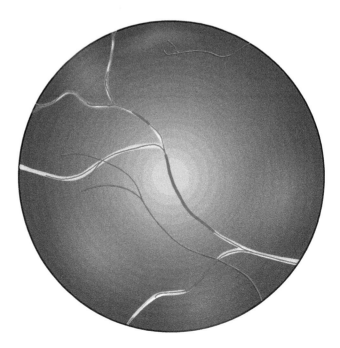

Figure 4.3 Sheathing of peripheral venules in intermediate uveitis.

Table 4.2 Summary of signs in intermediate uveitis

Examination of anterior vitreous	Examination of retina
Cells	Snowballs
Debris	Snowbank
Vitreous bands	Peripheral vasculitis with sheathing
	Neovascularisation
	Tractional retinal detachment (rare)

the vessel it implies an inflammatory process is taking place, although it must also be remembered that after the inflammation has settled the sheath takes weeks or even months to disperse and its continued presence is not necessarily indicative of ongoing inflammation.

These peripheral vessels can become, in severe cases, so inflamed that they become occluded and peripheral ischaemia results. This in turn can lead to **neovascularisation** and **vitreous traction** which in turn can cause a tractional **retinal detachment**. This is rare however and the intermediate uveitis that tends to present to eye casualty as a new patient will not have had time to develop neovascularisation, gliosis and traction, unless there was some factor which prevented the patient from attending despite symptoms for a long period of time. Likewise it is also possible for severe prolonged inflammation to result in an exudative retinal detachment but overall this is rare and at the first visit very rare indeed. So rare in fact that I am not going to highlight it in italics.

The main reason the vision becomes blurred in intermediate uveitis is the presence of cystoid macular oedema (CMO), which is much more common than with anterior uveitis. It is important to watch out for glaucoma and cataract, as with anterior uveitis, which can occur as a result of either the inflammation or the treatment. Last it is possible in severe inflammation that in addition to the macula the optic disc may become mildly swollen (Table 4.2).

Once a history and examination have been undertaken the time will have come to grade the severity of the condition and think about investigations.

PITFALLS

As with all uveitic patients it is important to consider and rule out other causes of cells, or material in the vitreous which can occasionally be confused with intermediate uveitis. Pigment cells, for example, also called tobacco dust, may be present in the vitreous following a rhegmatogenous retinal detachment, ocular uveal melanomas, or rarely in association with pigment dispersion. Similarly, red blood cells either as fresh blood, or altered blood, in the vitreous can occur with any of the multitude causes of a vitreous haemorrhage. While these causes are usually easy to distinguish from inflammation they should of course be considered, if only to be ruled out.

More sinisterly the vitreous gel can become infiltrated with malignant cells. The most important condition to beware of is primary intraocular lymphoma, a variant of primary central nervous system (CNS) lymphoma (Chapter 6). This rare condition is frequently misdiagnosed and mistreated as intermediate uveitis, and this does the patient no favours.

SEVERITY

Having examined the anterior chamber before proceeding to the anterior vitreous the ophthalmologist would already have noted any anterior chamber activity and measured the cells

Table 4.3 Grading vitreous haze as per the SUN classification

Grade	Description	Fundoscopy
0	Nil	Normal
1	Minimal	Debris present but posterior pole clear and crisp
2	Mild	Posterior pole slightly hazy
3	Moderate	Posterior pole very hazy
4	Marked	Disc and major vessels visible but only just
5	Severe	No fundal details visible

and flare appropriately. This is the same as in Chapter 3. The vitreitis grading is done by taking vitreous haze into consideration as per Table 4.3. The vitreous haze must be graded by binocular indirect ophthalmoscopy, using a 20-dioptre lens. Note that the degree of haze might be different when looking in different directions so it is graded by convention with regard to how clearly posterior pole details can be visualised.

There are also grading systems for vitreous cells that you may find in other texts, some of which require the antiquated Hruby lens to be used, but we do not advise the use of any of these systems as vitreous haze is by far the better indicator of inflammatory activity. It is important however to note the nature of the cell itself as anterior vitreous cells that are pigmented as opposed to being clear are far more likely to be older and of less immediate consequence.

Tip: **Measure the vitreous haze but do not attempt to measure vitreous cells.**

INVESTIGATIONS

The investigations that are carried out are dependent on the overall clinical picture. There are some authors who attempt to differentiate between two different subsets of intermediate uveitis – one in which there is substantial snowbanking and the other where there is not. The former is sometimes very unhelpfully called 'pars planitis' and investigated and treated differently to all other cases of intermediate uveitis but should a person ask where is the border between one and the other then the huge degree of overlap renders the whole exercise pointless. It is far better to consider the most common systemic associations, bearing in mind that 70% of cases are idiopathic, and asking clinical questions related to these with investigations only being undertaken if there are suggestive systemic symptoms.

The most common systemic associations are sarcoidosis, multiple sclerosis (MS), Lyme disease, tuberculosis (TB) and syphilis. Please bear in mind that the various causes will be of differing frequencies in various geographical locations. In India and Pakistan, for example the overwhelming cause will likely be TB, in the forests of rural Eastern Europe Lyme disease is more important and in northern sun-starved vitamin D-deprived Caucasian populations such as the Welsh, Irish and Scottish people multiple sclerosis is far more important. Immigration, travel and race must also be borne in mind as certain areas of London act as exclaves of the subcontinent and TB again becomes important. Bearing this in mind having routine tests that are performed as standard in any uveitic condition will certainly lead to confusion and disaster. What is the purpose of performing a serum angiotensin-converting enzyme (ACE) test if there are no suggestive symptoms of sarcoid whatsoever? If it is positive will you act on it? Table 4.4 suggests appropriate questions to ask when faced with a patient with intermediate uveitis.

If the patient answers negatively to any of these questions then we suggest no investigation be performed. If they answer positively then dig deeper to determine the exact symptoms and the

Table 4.4 Systemic associations of intermediate uveitis and suggested screening questions

Systemic disease	Screening question
Sarcoidosis	Have you had any cough, shortness of breath, any aches in your joints or lumps on the skin?
Multiple sclerosis	Have you had any weakness, numbness or tingling in any part of your body or any other neurological symptom? Have you noticed excessive fatigue?
Lyme disease	Do you enjoy walking, hiking or camping in the forest, near large animals such as horses or deer?
Tuberculosis (TB)	Have you been exposed to anyone with TB or visited areas where people have TB?
Syphilis	We ask everyone these questions as sometimes eye inflammation can be related to a sexually transmitted disease. How many people have you had sex with in the past 6 months and were they male, female or both? Did you have protected or unprotected sex and what kind of intercourse did you have? Have you ever paid for sex?

Table 4.5 Investigations for the five major systemic associations of intermediate uveitis

Systemic disease	Investigation
Sarcoidosis	Serum ACE and calcium, CXR
Multiple sclerosis	Neurology referral
Lyme disease	Referral to infectious disease specialist – Lyme serology is controversial due to low sensitivity and specificity
Tuberculosis	Quantiferon gold blood test, Mantoux and CXR
Syphilis	Treponemal serology

extent so that appropriate decision-making can take place. MS is a tricky one as 15% of patients with intermediate uveitis may develop this condition and patients with MS are 10 times more likely to develop intermediate uveitis in turn than those without. Nevertheless it is better not to investigate should the patient deny any neurological symptom whatsoever, though educated patients may search the Internet and ask about the association with MS in which case it is better to answer any question honestly. The investigations carried out for the above conditions are listed in Table 4.5.

Other rarer causes of intermediate uveitis such as cat scratch, toxoplasmosis and toxocariasis can be borne in mind though unless the clinical picture is indicative a routine question about each in a standard presentation is not necessary as otherwise the false-positive answers will start to rise and you will take so long assessing the patient that unnecessary clinic delays will occur. There is a tendency to investigate syphilis and TB together or not at all as one can mimic the other, and while we do not particularly endorse this view there are many who do. A computed tomography (CT) scan of the thorax is a more detailed test to look for sarcoidosis, but it should be a test that is considered and ordered by a respiratory physician rather than an ophthalmologist. A fundus fluorescein angiogram (FFA) is not usually very useful with intermediate uveitis, unless the diagnosis is in doubt or if peripheral ischaemia is a factor and laser therapy is planned.

CYSTOID MACULAR OEDEMA

CMO is much more common in intermediate uveitis than with anterior uveitis so we would advocate having a low threshold for performing this ocular coherence tomography (OCT) scanning. The mainstay of treatment is to prevent CMO from forming and to treat it if it does in a manner different to inflammation without macular fluid; thus the criteria for justifying an investigation are fulfilled. If fluid is present once then at all subsequent visits the patient should undergo an OCT scan, as this wondrous device can pick up fluid the naked ophthalmic eye at the slit lamp could never have and it provides an objective measurement that can be used to grade severity and measure improvement. You can however be misled by an over-reliance on OCT scanning as younger patients can have excellent retinal pigment epithelium (RPE) pump function so the only evidence of leakage might be on angiogram. That said, if the OCT is dry no action needs to be taken specifically for this other than controlling the inflammation.

WHY TREAT INTERMEDIATE UVEITIS?

Before treating any condition it is always worth asking 'why?'. By far the biggest reason is to prevent or treat CMO, which will blur the vision in the short term and if allowed to be present for more than a few months will permanently injure the fovea. Less importantly, and more rarely, peripheral ischaemia and neovascularisation may result in a tractional retinal detachment or a vitreous haemorrhage. A cataract may also form, necessitating the need for cataract surgery, and if spillover anterior uveitis is substantial posterior synechiae may form with all the attendant complications mentioned in the previous chapter. Lastly glaucoma may occur, though this is usually less of an issue than with primary anterior uveitis. After the inflammation is rendered quiet the eye must be monitored for recurrences, and should these be a problem maintenance therapy may need to be instituted. Unlike with anterior uveitis the eye is less symptomatic when inflamed and recurrences are far more common so follow-up becomes more important and absolute discharge less likely.

TREATMENT

As would be expected the treatment of intermediate uveitis is entirely dependent on the results of the investigations, if any had been done at all. Considering and then ruling out an infectious cause can be considered the first step. If an infectious cause was suspected and testing undertaken then the specific cause should be treated, and similarly for inflammatory causes. If testing for sarcoid returns positive results then referral to a chest physician is indicated in the event of the lungs being affected or a rheumatologist if there are multiple systems involved. If there are chest symptoms but the chest x-ray (CXR) is clear then consider a chest CT scan. The aim is to build enough evidence to be able to justify a referral to a chest physician. It is pointless sending an almost asymptomatic patient with normal ACE and CXR; they will either reject the referral or see the patient and say nothing needs to be done. The other systemic illnesses should be treated the same. If there are neurological symptoms make a note of them all and write to a neurologist so they can consider a magnetic resonance imaging (MRI) scan of the head to look for MS. As a general rule it is better for ophthalmologists not to order the MRI scan as the neurologist will be better able to have discussions with the patient based on the result, the probability of developing MS, potential treatments and prognosis than we are.

   If the patient tested positive for Lyme, a test which only should have been done if there had been a suggestive history and supporting evidence, then referral to a physician or infectious disease specialist is best. While ophthalmologists can and do treat Lyme, it must be remembered that this is a multi-system disease and we may not be the best-placed people to look at the dermatological, cardiac and neurological aspects of this potentially life-threatening condition. Likewise TB is best managed by a respiratory physician specialising in TB and a positive syphilis test will simply mean a referral to a genitourinary clinic. It should perhaps be noted here that there is a small but growing minority of patients with the symptomatology of chronic fatigue syndrome/myalgic encephalomyelitis (ME) who for reasons of perceived prejudice against this condition will seek a diagnosis of Lyme disease even though testing may prove negative, though a complicating factor of course is the ongoing positivity of tests weeks or years after the successful treatment of Lyme disease and their poor indicator of active disease.

Tip: If systemic associations are found refer the patient promptly to the relevant speciality – do not try and treat the patient yourself.

Systemic associations are important as they affect how intermediate uveitis is treated. Local therapy is the same whether the condition is idiopathic or related to a systemic condition, so long as the appropriate systemic therapy is also instituted. For example if a patient is on TB therapy, or doxycycline for Lyme, or having antibiotics for syphilis, the drop regimens and local therapy techniques are the same, but if no systemic treatment is undertaken when say TB or syphilis is present then giving steroid injections can make things potentially worse. In cases where systemic immunosuppression is needed missing an infection such as TB can be life threatening for the patient. If systemic immunosuppression is needed in inflammatory conditions such as sarcoid it is best to coordinate this with the respiratory physicians or the rheumatologists involved as they might have been considering the same. With infectious conditions it is better to ask the treating physician when it is safe to institute systemic immunosuppressant medication, though by and large this is a problem with TB rather than syphilis or Lyme.

Table 4.6 describes a treatment regime for a patient with intermediate uveitis without CMO. Note that prednisolone acetate 1% (Pred Forte) may also be substituted for Maxidex.

The observant will note that Table 4.6 is similar to Table 3.5 in the previous chapter on anterior uveitis, with the only difference being that there is significantly less need for cyclopentolate. With intermediate uveitis a drop regime is particularly well suited for treating patients with no systemic manifestation, or as a short-term boost to treat an ocular flare-up of an otherwise treated and well-controlled systemic condition. Following cataract surgery topical therapy is more effective due to enhanced penetration through long-term treatment. While this is successful for most people it may become burdensome in older patients. Table 4.7 indicates the therapies that may be needed in certain circumstances.

Table 4.6 A treatment regime for a patient with intermediate uveitis without CMO

Drop frequency	Duration
Dexamethasone (Maxidex) hourly	1 week
Cyclopentolate 1% tds (if needed)	1 week then stop
Dexamethasone (Maxidex) every other hour	1 week
Qds	1 week
Tds	1 week
Bd	1 week
Od	1 week

Table 4.7 Therapies that may be needed to control intermediate uveitis

Severity	Treatment
Inflammation without CMO	Regime as per Table 4.6
Inflammation with CMO	As above plus topical ketorolac (acular) qds for 6 weeks
Inflammation with CMO despite topical treatment	Orbital floor injection of 40 mg triamcinolone acetonide (kenalog) in 1 mL
Still no response	Intravitreal steroid – 0.1 mL of kenalog (4 mg) or Ozurdex implant
Still no response or bilateral CMO	Oral prednisolone (if systemic condition allows) 60 mg rapid taper
Inflammation recurs	Slower taper or other immunomodulatory agents

An **orbital floor injection** of kenalog can be done in the following manner, having obtained patient consent:

1. This injection can be done in the clinic room without needing a clean room. Shake the vial of kenalog well.
2. Draw up 1 mL of kenalog into a 1 mL syringe using a green needle (21 gauge). Using a filtered needle or a smaller needle will result in failure due to immediate blockage.
3. Swap the green needle for a long orange needle (25 gauge) and expel the air.
4. Wipe an alcohol swab along the lower lid to sterilise the skin.
5. Ask the patient to look up and at a point at the junction between the medial two thirds and lateral third of the lower eyelid directly above the inferior orbital margin and perpendicular to the skin insert the needle.
6. Advance the needle along the orbital floor while asking the patient to look up and down, left and right in order to be sure the globe is not engaged.
7. You may hit the bone while you advance the needle; should this occur do not worry, angle the needle slightly upwards and continue to advance.
8. When the needle is fully inserted inject the 1 mL of steroid and withdraw the needle.
9. Massage site with tissue.

An orbital floor injection is usually safe and problem free with an easy learning curve but does involve a sharp needle. This might be an issue with an anxious patient or an inexperienced clinician. In these cases a sub-Tenon's injection may be preferred as this involves using a blunt needle called a sub-Tenon's cannula. A **sub-Tenon's injection** is performed as follows:

1. Lie the patient down on an examination couch. A clean room is again not needed. Shake the vial of kenalog well.
2. Draw up 1 mL of kenalog into a 1 mL syringe using a green needle (21 gauge). Using a filtered needle or a smaller needle will result in failure due to immediate blockage.
3. Swap the green needle for a sub-Tenon's cannula and expel the air.
4. Apply a minim of oxybuprocaine topical anaesthetic to the conjunctival sac of the eye to be injected, followed by a drop of 5% iodine.
5. Insert a lid speculum and ask the patient to look 'up and out' as the injection site will be in the inferonasal quadrant.
6. Grasp the conjunctiva and Tenon's capsule approximately 10 mm or so inferonasally with a toothed pair of forceps and pull them gently away from the globe. Using a pair of curved scissors make a cut in the tissue pulled forward.
7. While keeping the traction with the forceps insert the closed pair of scissors into the cut and curve them around so that the curve follows the shape of the globe. Do this until the

scissors are vertical; a 'pop' can be felt as the scissors gently pass through the adhesions present at the equator.

8. Withdraw the scissors and insert the curved sub-Tenon's cannula, again following the curve of the globe, and when fully inserted and vertical inject the 1 mL of triamcinolone.
9. There should not be much reflux. If this is not the case, try and pull the cannula slightly away from the globe to create a space in which to inject.
10. Withdraw the cannula, let go with the forceps and remove the speculum.

Kenalog may be injected **intravitreally** as well as along the orbit floor and under Tenon's capsule, but note that this is not a licensed use of triamcinolone and it might be difficult to justify its use when a licenced alternative, Ozurdex, is also available. The cost differential is worthy of note in this case however, with Ozurdex being much more expensive than triamcinolone. Any intravitreal injection will need to take place in a clean room. Figure 4.4 demonstrates an orbital floor injection being performed. Intravitreal steroid can last up to 4 months while a sub-Tenon's or orbital floor injection can last around 3 months which makes it an impractical option for long-term management. Rather, it is for treating acute exacerbations, particularly when CMO is an issue. As well as with all the usual ocular side effects of steroids, such as a rise in intraocular pressure and cataract formation, there are additional possible local problems that can occur following an orbital floor injection of steroid such as haemorrhage and ecchymosis, short-term diplopia if an extraocular muscle is damaged and skin pigment loss at the site of the injection in darker-skinned races. There are even rare reports of globe perforation. Young females in particular may be troubled by a fullness of the lower lid crease which creates a slight cosmetic issue that occurs as a result of trauma to the orbital septum.

Table 4.8 indicates a rapid tapering regime for oral prednisolone. A slower tapering course may be indicated and if so will be dependent on the dosage which the patient was on when the disease became active again and is specific to the patient. For example if the patient reactivated when the dose was reduced from 20 to 10 mg of oral prednisolone then the slow tapering will start from 20 mg once control has been established via Table 4.8. The slow tapering can be organised over weeks or months but getting the patient to 7.5 mg/day of prednisolone, or less,

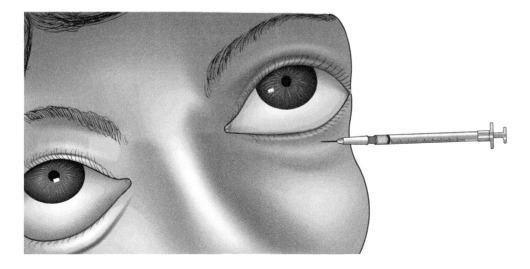

Figure 4.4 An orbital floor injection being performed.

Table 4.8 A rapid tapering regime for oral prednisolone

Dose of prednisolone/day	Duration
60 mg	1 week
40 mg	1 week
30 mg	1 week
20 mg	1 week
10 mg	1 week
5 mg	1 week

is the name of the game. If this is not possible without a flare-up occurring then immunosuppression may be needed (see Chapter 8).

The purpose of the **rapid tapering regime** is to establish rapid control and allow for a quick withdrawal once the eye is quiet allowing topical treatment to be more effective. This can be compared to a riot in a prison where the normal contingent of guards are not enough to control the riotous inmates but once the prisoners are back in their cells courtesy of a flying visit by the riot squad they become much more manageable. If the prison immediately erupts into violence as soon as the riot squad leaves, then it must be acknowledged that there may be a need for some permanent presence of riot police. That topical therapy alone may not cut the mustard, in our analogy.

The **slow tapering regime** as mentioned starts from the step above when the inflammation recurred on the rapid tapering regime and can descend at 5 mg per week, 5 mg every other week, 2.5 mg every other week, 2.5 mg every 4 weeks or 2.5 mg step-downs at even longer intervals. There is generally not much point in descending in aliquots of 1 mg in this condition or indeed the vast majority of any uveitis condition as the only purpose of this is to convince the patient and the ophthalmologist that they are 'doing something'. Should the eye flare up again at a lower dose then an even slower tapering regime from the step above can be employed and the patient maintained on a dose of 7.5 mg of daily prednisolone for 6 months prior to an attempt to further reduce should the eye be quiet. The aim is to keep the eye quiet for at least 2 years at a dose of 7.5 mg prednisolone or less before attempting to stop the medication altogether. Should the inflammation rebound at this dose a steroid sparing immunosuppressive agent must be considered. There are numerous voodoo myths and legends about the immune system 'resetting' after 2 years of quiescence, but despite the lack of overwhelming evidence there is some logic to it, and even if there was no logic, there must be a plan and something to aim for. Should the eye flare up necessitating doses of greater than 7.5 mg of prednisolone to keep the eye quiet a steroid sparing agent will be needed. See Chapter 8 for more information about corticosteroid precautions and patient management plans. Chapter 3 discusses drop tapering and maintenance regimes for anterior uveitis and this holds true for intermediate uveitis as well.

Should a patient, particularly an elderly patient, develop an intermediate uveitis which does not appear to have a systemic association and which responds transiently if at all to steroids always consider the possibility of **intraocular lymphoma** (see Chapter 6). Should this suspicion arise order an MRI of the head to look for intracranial lymphoma, and should this be positive refer your patient to the oncology team for management. Should the MRI be normal a referral to an ocular oncologist is indicated. Do not ask a vitreoretinal colleague to perform a diagnostic vitrectomy if based outside one of the major ocular oncology centres as this specialist work requires specialist pathology services, and transporting the fluid independent of the patient to the specialist centre is more likely to result in false-negatives. The best transport container is the human eye.

Should a patient with intermediate uveitis develop a **cataract** which needs extraction then they need to be covered with topical steroids, as with anterior uveitis, before the operation. As with anterior uveitis it is important to wait until the eye has been quiet for 3 months before proceeding, otherwise it will be a bad time all round for the patient and the ophthalmologist. A popular choice of pre-operative steroid is Maxidex four times a day (qds) for a week followed by the regime in Table 3.5 after the operation, as well as a week of topical post-operative antibiotic cover such as ofloxacin qds. Should the patient have needed oral steroids in the past or is on a maintenance dose of steroids at present then 40 mg of oral prednisolone for 5 days pre-operatively followed by the regime in Table 4.8 works well. Obviously if the patient is on maintenance oral steroid then stopping at the usual dose rather than weaning off completely is the best plan.

In the unlikely event that the patient develops peripheral **neovascularisation** then laser to ischaemic retina is indicated, preferably preceded by a wide-field angiogram if available. If an epiretinal membrane or tractional detachment starts to occur then a referral to a vitreoretinal colleague may be indicated.

FOLLOW-UP

This is entirely dependent on the activity of the disease and the treatment the patient is on. If on topical steroids then 4–6 weekly gaps are appropriate if the patient is improving. If on oral steroids it might be prudent to have shorter intervals, at least initially, of 2–4 weeks. After injection of orbital floor or intraocular triamcinolone then a visit to look for a possible rise in intraocular pressure at the 4-week mark is a must. If the eye is stable off all treatment then 3-monthly follow-up for a year is prudent to look for the early signs of reactivation, although the educational status of your patient may influence this decision, and you may be able to discharge them earlier if you can rely on them to get back in touch if they run into difficulty. If they are stable on a maintenance dose of topical or oral steroid then follow-up intervals of between 3 and 6 months in perpetuity are indicated. If a steroid-sparing agent has been deployed the follow-up will be entirely dependent on the drug (see Chapter 8).

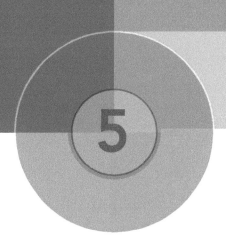

Posterior uveitis

We come now to the most confusing aspect of the entire field of inflammatory eye disease. Ophthalmologists in training usually become used to seeing patients with anterior uveitis very early on in their careers due to their sheer numbers and by the end of their training have seen enough intermediate uveitis cases to know roughly what investigations to order and how to treat it, at least in the short term. Posterior uveitis, making up to 7% of all cases of uveitis, though these figures vary depending on the eye department in which you work, is the type that causes ophthalmologists to lose sleep and to panic when faced with their first ever case. This is because of all the variants of uveitis, posterior uveitis has the possibility to blind a patient within days or even hours if left untreated and where the treatments, much like those seen in the *House* TV series starring Hugh Laurie, can either cure the patient or make their condition much worse. Also, compared with either anterior or intermediate uveitis the list of probable diagnoses here is much longer. While all this might be true the subject is in fact simpler than people assume and simpler than the mighty tomes of uveitis make it. Let us start at first principles.

WHAT IS POSTERIOR UVEITIS?

To get to this point by definition we must have already explored the anterior chamber and vitreous. If there had been a lot of inflammation anteriorly and less if any in the vitreous then we would already suspect that the posterior pole and fundus would be quiet. If there had been no or only mild anterior chamber activity but more in the vitreous then our suspicions would already have been raised that a posterior uveitis is a possibility. Posterior uveitis is present when the source of the inflammation is located in the retina or choroid. So by definition there must be some evidence of change on the fundus along with inflammation. The only fundal change allowed with anterior uveitis is cystoid macular oedema (CMO) and the only posterior pole changes allowed with intermediate uveitis are CMO and a mildly swollen optic disc.

Posterior uveitis is uveitis which is accompanied by changes to the fundus and in which the source of the inflammation is the retina or choroid.

There must be evidence of change. You may have to look for it with a thorough search but there must be evidence. Posterior uveitis is a large umbrella term and many conditions exist under it, some aggressive and some very subtle. They may be so subtle that to the ophthalmologist examining the patient all appears well and the abnormality can only be detected by optical coherence tomography (OCT) scanning, or fundus fluorescein angiography (FFA), or visual field test (VFT), or even on electrophysiological studies such as an electroretinogram (ERG) or other electrodiagnostic tests (EDT); but they must be present. The sequence of events that would have taken place to get to this point would have been as follows:

1. The anterior segment is explored and there may or may not be signs of inflammation discovered.
2. The vitreous is examined and there may or may not be signs of inflammation discovered. If anterior signs were discovered and the vitreous is involved the examination of the fundus is what then determines whether this is an intermediate or a posterior uveitis.
3. If there were thus far no signs of inflammation there is some abnormality of the fundus which indicates an inflammatory process. If there is a vitritis and if the signs are only very peripheral then this is an intermediate uveitis, but if there are signs more posteriorly then this is a posterior uveitis.

Once we have established that a posterior uveitis is present the huge list of differential diagnoses can be broken down into easily manageable chunks but the first step is ensuring that it is a posterior uveitis. There are conditions which cause scars and masses and vascular problems and all kinds of abnormalities of the fundus, in fact a large portion of the field of ophthalmology, but are not indicative of posterior uveitis. If there is anterior uveitis present but the vitreous is clear it is very unlikely that noticing a fundal abnormality will make this the source of the inflammation. If there is a vascular occlusion however in the face of dense vitritis but only moderate anterior uveitis then a posterior uveitis is very probably present. You can never be sure of course but the state of the vitreous is a big clue. It might be that as well as the anterior uveitis the vitreous is so inflamed that the posterior pole is not very visible and the examining ophthalmologist cannot be sure if there is a fundal component but this is a situation termed 'panuveitis' and is dealt with in Chapter 6.

HISTORY

It might be best to consider posterior uveitis a more aggressive version of intermediate uveitis with regard to the presentation of the patient. Unlike anterior uveitis rather than pain and photophobia patients tend to have **floaters, blurred or distorted vision, visual field disturbances** or **photopsia**, where flashing lights are seen. Table 5.1 illustrates how the three forms of uveitis tend to present.

What can confuse the matter is that certain forms of posterior uveitis are very aggressive and can rapidly spread to a full panuveitis where pain and photophobia then become an issue, although the condition may have started as a posterior uveitis. Some forms of posterior uveitis

Table 5.1 How history can help differentiate between the three forms of uveitis

Anterior uveitis	Intermediate uveitis	Posterior uveitis
Photophobia	Blurred vision	Blurred vision
Pain	Floaters	Floaters
Blurred vision	Asymptomatic	Visual field disturbances
		Photopsia

never do this, though it highlights again the importance of a full dilated examination in all cases of suspected uveitis.

Tip: A full dilated examination of the fundus in all cases of uveitis is a must.

It is important to establish the timeline of the symptoms in the history and whether the symptoms have been persistent (present for longer than 3 months – see Chapter 1) or whether they have been sudden and dramatic. Previous attacks or episodes are also important to note here, as are systemic symptoms. As there are myriad conditions that cause posterior uveitis it is impossible to ask after every single systemic association for every condition before the patient has been examined. Here it is prudent to ask before examining the patient a broad question about any past medical problems and then use the examination to hone in on specific symptoms that are then much more useful in differentiating between different groups of conditions. Don't ask about mouth ulcers or genital ulcers, for example, unless your examination suggests Behçet's disease might be a possibility.

CLASSIFICATION BY EXAMINATION

The first thing to determine is whether the patient has an active potentially sight-threatening pathology, and if the history is of profound visual loss happening over days rather than weeks or months then this is a possibility. If this is not the case the second question is to ask which of the long list of remaining pathologies might be at work. This depends a lot on a view of the posterior pole and if this is not possible due to the level of inflammation then certain basic principles need to be followed. This is explained in detail in Chapter 6. Let us look at how we can answer these two important questions in a logical manner.

Question 1: Does the patient have an active potentially sight-threatening pathology?

Any condition, within reason, can with sufficient time blind a patient. What we are mostly concerned with here is whether the condition is particularly aggressive to the extent that inaction or incorrect action at the first visit will result in harm. These conditions by definition will have an acute history of a few days up to a week or so and looking for these conditions first starts to make the long lists of differentials manageable. Table 5.2 contains a list of conditions that are acute, dangerous and which you should consider first on your diagnostic algorithm when faced with posterior uveitis. Notice that they are all infectious conditions, though a note of caution here states that Behçet's disease may present acutely with white patches of retina with adjacent haemorrhage and may be considered here as well if this is the mode of presentation. It is considered in more detail later in this chapter.

Table 5.2 Conditions to consider first in a patient with an acute posterior uveitis

Condition	Examination
Acute retinal necrosis (ARN)	White patches of retina with vasculitis
Infectious endophthalmitis	Very blurred view with clumps of inflammatory debris in the vitreous
Toxoplasmosis – certain lesions	White patch of retina next to pigmented retinal lesion
Behçet's disease	Small white patches of retinal infiltrate with adjacent haemorrhage

The first clue as to what is going on will depend on what you see at first glance of the fundus. If the view is obscured by a huge amount of vitreous inflammation with severe anterior chamber involvement you must try hard to see the retina. That will include looking at the periphery as the view can be clearer here, or lying the patient down on an examination table and using an indirect ophthalmoscope to examine the fundus as the optics are such that the view can be clearer. A Superfield or 90D Volk lens is the best lens to view the periphery at the slit lamp. If the retina is visualised it can be said to be normal or abnormal. If it is abnormal look for white patches or pigmented patches and these are either present or absent. The history will be a guide as well:

- Have you had any recent eye surgery? Are you unwell, or have you been unwell in the past week? Ask about any recent febrile illnesses, any cough, fevers, symptoms of a urinary tract infection or the presence of a hot swollen joint. Is there a history of current or recent intravenous cannulation? Is there a possibility of intravenous drug abuse? Have you had recent or past cardiac valve replacement surgery? If so then infectious endophthalmitis is a strong possibility if the view is blurred but the retina you do see seems normal.
- Have you ever had an inflammation of the eye before which caused your vision to become blurred like this? If so then a reactivation of toxoplasmosis may be a possibility. Certain **toxoplasmosis** lesions if located close to the **fovea, optic disc** or **arcade vessels** need immediate treatment to prevent permanent damage to vision.

If extensive white patches of retina are seen in an acute setting the diagnosis must be acute retinal necrosis until proven otherwise. The intraocular pressure is an important clue directing the ophthalmologist to a potentially sight-threatening cause of posterior uveitis as toxoplasmosis characteristically presents in the acute phase with a **raised intraocular pressure** due to concurrent trabeculitis preventing egress of fluid from the eye, while acute retinal necrosis is typically normotensive.

If the patient does not have an immediately sight-threatening condition then the second question can be asked.

Question 2: What else could be the cause of the posterior uveitis?

There are multiple ways to break down the remaining list of differential diagnoses into manageable chunks. Many texts divide by inflammatory or infective causes, or retinitis or choroiditis, and while these may be useful in a pure Linnaean sense they are not useful distinctions for ophthalmologists. It is better to follow an algorithm where we first remove the immediate sight-threatening conditions and then classify what is left. The first obvious question is: Are there dots/spots on the fundus?

Are there dots/spots all over the fundus? By this I mean round or ovoid lesions scattered over the fundus in varying numbers, not a patch here or a mass there but a general smattering of spots. The answer is either yes or no.

If yes, then Table 5.3 will help us narrow down our differential diagnoses. If no, or there is something else of much greater significance occurring, we must pass on to the next question below.

Table 5.3 starts with the most obvious spots at the top and the most difficult to see at the bottom. The following adage is funny because it is true – 'If the eye casualty doctor diagnoses MEWDS (multiple evanescent white dot syndrome) there can be no MEWDS present'. Much is made of the fact that some conditions are unilateral, notably MEWDS, and others are bilateral, notably acute posterior multifocal placoid pigment epitheliopathy (APMPPE), but

Table 5.3 Fundal dots/spots and their associated conditions

Description of fundal dot/spot	Suggested cause of posterior uveitis
Easy to see large spots a disc diameter or more with variable degrees of pigmentation	Acute posterior multifocal placoid pigment epitheliopathy (APMPPE)
Easy to see deep spots less than a disc diameter of various pigmentation all around the periphery with peri-papillary scarring	Multifocal choroiditis with panuveitis
Easy to see deep spots less than half a disc diameter of various pigmentation limited to the posterior pole and macula	Punctate inner choroidopathy
Easy to see deep spots a quarter of a disc diameter in lines or groups without inflammation	Presumed ocular histoplasmosis syndrome
Less easy to see spots yellow in nature around a quarter or less of a disc diameter scattered all over the fundus lacking pigment	Birdshot chorioretinopathy
Less easy to see spots yellow in nature around a quarter or less of a disc diameter scattered all over the fundus with varying amounts of pigment	Sarcoidosis
Very difficult to see grey spots less than a tenth of a disc diameter at the posterior pole	Multiple evanescent white dot syndrome (MEWDS)
Any of the above	Syphilis

there are exceptions to these rules so they are not stressed here. If the patient falls into one of the above categories go below to the relevant section for more information.

Question 3: Is there a vasculitis present?

Many forms of uveitis can be associated with a vasculitis but what is meant here is that the most obvious feature when looking at the fundus is a vasculitis. This is an inflammation of blood vessels in which there is sheathing. This is a coating of inflammatory exudate which can vary between a very subtle gloss similar to what might be imagined if the vessel was covered with a condom, to an appearance similar to tree twigs covered in winter snow or surrounded by a dense layer of candle wax. The inflamed vessel can then become occluded resulting in ischaemic signs such as cotton wool spots, microaneurysms, dot or blot haemorrhages and neovascularisation.

If a vasculitis is the most obvious thing seen when looking at the fundus then the next step is to see whether the form of vasculitis present helps us diagnostically or not. Note that though there is much overlap there are specific presentations that suggest specific diagnoses. Table 5.4 illustrates how looking at the vessels can help differentiate between the common differential diagnoses. By following our suggested algorithm if acute retinal necrosis is present or birdshot chorioretinopathy

Table 5.4 Looking at the retinal vessels to aid diagnosis of posterior uveitis

Vascular sign	Suggested cause of posterior uveitis
Branch retinal vein occlusion	Behçet's disease
Periphlebitis – inflammation of the veins	TB, sarcoidosis
Branch retinal artery occlusion	Polyarteritis nodosa, Susac syndrome, cat scratch disease
Arteritis – inflammation of the arteries	Idiopathic retinal vasculitis with aneurysms and neuroretinitis (IRVAN)
Any of the above	TB, syphilis

then these would have been detected before now so the list of differentials is somewhat lessened and has become more manageable, hence the low number of diagnoses in Table 5.4.

It must be noted that there is no systemic association in the majority of cases of vasculitis though Table 5.4 describes particular conditions that are very strongly linked to particular fundal appearances. There is a huge list of conditions, some not uncommon and some vanishingly rare, that can cause retinal vasculitis. These conditions, including Churg-Strauss syndrome, granulomatosis with polyangiitis (GPA – Wegener's granulomatosis), Whipple's disease and Rift valley fever virus, are so numerous that considering each separately is not useful. A better approach is to see if the appearances fit into Table 5.4 and if so asking appropriate questions about these conditions. If however it is simply a case of posterior uveitis with a vasculitis which is not dramatic then asking about any systemic conditions, skin complaints or recent illnesses is best and if the patient denies any of these then it is mostly pointless to ask the ten thousand questions it would take to drill down into every possible cause of retinal vasculitis that exists. Many textbooks exist with tables of conditions that cause arteritis, phlebitis, ischaemia, occlusive disease and more, with each box containing many conditions and usually the same conditions as in the other boxes.

A note of caution must be sounded here as lymphoma and leukaemia can cause vascular issues that can mimic a severe vasculitis. If the picture is severe in both eyes with multiple signs of ischaemia but no obvious inflammation it is prudent to perform appropriate investigations to look for these conditions, mainly in the form of a full blood count (FBC), before referring the patient to a haematologist if any suggestive abnormality is found.

By now we will have winnowed out the severe immediately sight-threatening conditions, the conditions with spots and the conditions with significant vasculitis as a main feature. Should the patient have none of these things the next question to ask is whether there is any obvious fundal lesion present that stands out.

Question 4: Is there a fundal lesion present as part of the posterior uveitis syndrome that does not fit into the above categories?

There are specific conditions that do not present primarily with dots, spots or vasculitis, though they may have some element of these pathologies, but have other very useful distinguishing features. Table 5.5 outlines specific conditions that cause posterior uveitis and their hallmark features.

It must be remembered that fundal scars from innumerable causes can occur which are totally unrelated to the cause of a posterior uveitis. As previously mentioned this umbrella of posterior uveitis is large and contains many diagnoses. Some conditions have abnormalities that are rarely if ever associated with any actual uveitis. Presumed ocular histoplasmosis

Table 5.5 Causes of posterior uveitis that have specific hallmark features

Hallmark feature	Suggested cause of posterior uveitis
Pigmented patch of retina with white fluffy patch at one margin	Toxoplasmosis
Peripheral mass with fibroglial traction	Toxocariasis
Exudative retinal detachment with or without nodules or spots a tenth of the disc diameter across	Sympathetic ophthalmia or Vogt–Koyanagi–Harada syndrome
Plaque of scarring extending from the disc along the vessels in a pincer movement around the fovea	Serpiginous choroiditis
Extensive scarring throughout the fundus	Progressive subretinal fibrosis and uveitis syndrome, or severe APMPPE
Macular star formation with optic disc swelling	Cat scratch disease

syndrome (POHS) by definition has no signs of any uveitis present. Punctate inner choroidopathy (PIC) almost never has detectable inflammation present on examination, though ancillary testing with FFA may reveal some. We next come to the last question we ask in determining the cause of a posterior uveitis, a question which after the previous questions will only apply to people with symptoms but no apparent abnormality.

Question 5: Is there a hidden cause of posterior uveitis present?

If we return to Table 5.1, where we compare the presentation of posterior and intermediate uveitis, it can be seen that the main differences between the two are the photopsia and field defects that can be present in posterior uveitis. We now enter the strange category of such patients where at first glance all seems well with the fundus and the abnormalities can only be found by further testing or scrupulous examination. Table 5.6 demonstrates the main causes of posterior uveitis symptoms where the diagnosis is not immediately obvious.

This is one way of many to approach the diagnosis of posterior uveitis. It is only meant as a guide to help rapidly focus the mind on lists of potential differential diagnoses that are small enough to be able to handle with ease. Some texts differentiate inflammatory from infective aetiologies but while this differentiation is of course of supreme importance these conditions can present quite similarly so it is only useful in the treatment rather than the diagnostic side of things. It again must be remembered that in the majority of cases there is no condition found to be causative and the posterior uveitis is then termed 'idiopathic'. It also must be remembered that there are myriad case reports of many stressors, including drugs, that are associated with posterior uveitis. Much of the work of differentiating one condition from another is of relatively little value as the treatment, in the majority of cases immunosuppression in one form or another, is the same. We present here the minimum differentiation which must be done in order to correctly treat the patient and save sight. Before we return to the algorithm in detail let us recap the questions that we ask, in the correct order:

Question 1: Does the patient have an active potentially sight-threatening pathology?
Question 2: What else could be the cause of the posterior uveitis? Are there dots or spots all over the fundus?

Table 5.6 The seemingly normal fundus in posterior uveitis syndromes and how to detect the abnormality

Symptom	Investigation and abnormality	Suggested cause
Photopsia, temporal scotoma	Visual field tests show enlarged blind spot, relative afferent pupillary defect	Acute idiopathic blind spot enlargement
Photopsia, acute scotomata	Visual field tests show loss in affected area, OCT demonstrates outer retinal abnormalities, fundus autofluorescence demonstrates abnormal area	Acute zonal occult outer retinopathy
Central scotoma	OCT demonstrates outer retinal abnormalities. Fundus autofluorescence demonstrates abnormal area	Acute macular neuroretinopathy
Photopsia, blurred vision, acute central scotoma	Visual field tests show central loss Electrodiagnostic tests are characteristic	Cancer-associated retinopathy
Photopsia	Visual field tests show peripheral loss Electrodiagnostic tests are characteristic	Melanoma-associated retinopathy

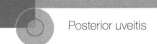

Question 3: Is there a vasculitis present?

Question 4: Is there a fundal lesion present as part of the posterior uveitis syndrome that does not fit into the above categories?

Question 5: Is there a hidden cause of posterior uveitis present?

Now let us go through this algorithm in detail.

DOES THE PATIENT HAVE POTENTIALLY SIGHT-THREATENING PATHOLOGY?

As mentioned all inflammatory conditions can become sight threatening if left long enough but here we examine three conditions where immediate action is necessary: acute retinal necrosis, infectious endophthalmitis and certain toxoplasmosis lesions.

ACUTE RETINAL NECROSIS

This condition is rare but devastating. It is the one thing not to miss as doing so will cause sight loss potentially within hours of the missed opportunity for intervention. It is the number one reason why uveitis specialists are called to give expert witness evidence in court with the classic scenario involving a patient treated for anterior uveitis in error as the ophthalmologist did not dilate the pupils to look at the fundi. The incidence rate of acute retinal necrosis (ARN) in the United Kingdom is around 0.6/million/year, suggesting that Wales, for example, should expect only two new cases of the disease each year on average.

There are two main viruses that cause this condition: the varicella zoster virus (VZV) and the herpes simplex virus (HSV). While classically this condition occurs in healthy patients being immunocompromised does pose a risk factor though cytomegalovirus (CMV) then becomes more important and the clinical presentation alters significantly. In fact the difference is so pronounced and incidence so much rarer again that it will be discussed separately, though there is some overlap. We will assume for this discussion that takes place in non-immunosuppressed patients. The age range in which it has been documented to occur is large at 13–85 years and although it is said that there are two peaks in which younger patients are more likely to have HSV as a cause and older patients VZV this does not alter anything clinically. While ARN is usually unilateral at presentation if left untreated the second eye can become involved in up to a third of patients. Table 5.7 demonstrates classic history and examination findings in ARN, while Figure 5.1 shows what the fundus of such a patient would look like.

Table 5.7 Symptoms and signs of ARN

Symptom	Sign
Decreased vision	Anterior chamber cells and flare
Floaters	Keratic precipitates
Ocular pain	Vitritis – may be severe
Photophobia	Peripheral white patches of retina with well-demarcated border
	Retinal arteritis
	Optic nerve swelling

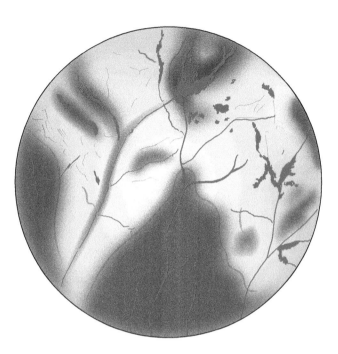

Figure 5.1 Funduscopic view of a patient with ARN.

The white patches of necrotic retina are the most important pathology to see in ARN and by definition they must be present. The actual configuration can vary from a small patch in one location to multiple patches with salients and panhandles extending posteriorly. Also by definition there will be vitritis present and this can be so severe as to limit the view of the fundus entirely. The anterior chamber can be heavily involved in such cases which highlights the importance of looking at the posterior segment in all cases of anterior uveitis. The affected area of retina tends to spread circumferentially first but progression is rapid and devastating. Fine pigmented keratic precipitates may be present, but occasionally they may be granulomatous.

Although the diagnosis is clinical, we recommend getting a virological diagnosis in all cases for several reasons. There is a saying at Moorfields that one can 'never regret getting a tap, but often regret not getting a tap'. This is particularly so if the condition does not respond to treatment. Identifying the virus can also guide therapy, and provide prognostic information as the prognosis is worse with VZV. If the clinical features are typical then we recommend an anterior chamber (AC) tap as the diagnostic yield is good. For typical cases we recommend an AC tap and intravitreal foscarnet – 2.4 mg in 0.1 mL, plus oral valaciclovir cover.

If the diagnosis is in doubt, then you are best advised obtaining vitreous biopsy performed by your vitreoretinal colleague. A controlled core vitrectomy with a vitreous cutter is far superior to a needle tap, which in any case is unlikely to give you the yield you need for all the tests. In addition, the typical ARN patient, if young, does not have a posterior vitreous detachment and you do not want to increase the already high rates of rhegmatogenous retinal detachment by pulling on the vitreous. Chapter 2 tells you how to perform an AC tap. A routine FBC is a useful tool in order to rule out any obvious immune system issues if there are none known, though the patient may be taking immunosuppressants for other systemic conditions. It is always wise to have a low threshold for testing for HIV.

The treatment of ARN is as shown in Table 5.8. Please note that these antivirals can cause renal dysfunction. Always get a baseline urea and electrolyte test. If the patient is known to have significant renal disease urgent advice from the renal team is advised as in these cases the effective, as well as the toxic dose of antiviral can be surprisingly small.

Topical steroids are used to treat anterior uveitis, along with topical cyclopentolate 1% in line with the regime suggested in Table 2.5 of Chapter 2. The use of oral steroids is controversial and hence they have not been included in Table 5.8. The benefits of oral steroids include a more rapidly clearing vitreous though the drawback is a potentially increased viral replication rate which could permanently harm vision. If the decision is made to use oral prednisolone a short regime of 40 mg for a week, 30 mg for a week, 20 mg for a week and 10 mg for a week is recommended. Steroid injections around or into the eye are **never** recommended.

Another controversial area is that of the usefulness of **barrier laser**. If the affected area is relatively small, well contained, the vitreous is not as hazy as it usually is and the anterior border is accessible then a barrier of laser around the edge of the necrotic lesion can reduce the chances of a subsequent retinal detachment. The truth of the matter is that the risk of a detachment in such a case would have been low anyway and with the high-risk detachment cases the affected area is usually so extensive and the vitreous so hazy that it would be a punishing task for both ophthalmologist and patient to laser around the whole area. In the acute phase it is better to leave things be, and this might also apply after the infection has settled.

The above describes clinically obvious ARN but there are variants of this alluded to above: progressive outer retinal necrosis (PORN) and CMV retinitis. These conditions exist in immunosuppressed states, classically HIV infection with low CD4 counts of less than 50 cells per mm^3. A grey area exists where patients may be immunocompromised for other less devastating reasons where the presentation of ARN may be more confusing than it normally is.

After a week of treatment there should be some observable signs of clinical improvement. There will be no extension of existing lesions or development of new ones and shortly afterwards the areas of necrosis will begin to look thickened. Two weeks after treatment has commenced the affected areas of retina will begin scar formation. If this is not the case the diagnosis will need to be reconsidered and if a tap had not been performed initially now will be the time that this is recommended. Other causes of retinitis such as toxoplasmosis, syphilis or Behçet's disease will now need to be considered. If the ARN worsens on treatment despite a virologically proven diagnosis then consider lack of drug compliance, an unexpected immunosuppressed state such as HIV positivity or drug resistance. If the latter is suspected, though rare, then the addition of oral valganciclovir can save the day as this is active against HSV and VZV as well as CMV.

PORN, a rather unfortunate acronym, is what results when ARN occurs in the context of severe immunosuppression, in that the virus involved is VZV (or HSV but much more rarely than in ARN, not that it matters) but the immune response is entirely lacking. There is no inflammation to cause pain so the presentation is usually with rapidly falling visual acuity in

Table 5.8 Treatment of ARN

First line	Oral valaciclovir 2 g three times a day (tds) for 2 weeks, then 1 g tds 6 weeks, then 500 mg tds 2 weeks
Second line	Intravenous acyclovir 10 mg/kg tds for 10–14 days, followed by switch to oral valaciclovir 1 g tds 6 weeks and taper as per above
If there is no improvement after 48 hours, or at presentation the uveitis is severe	Intravitreal foscarnet 2.4 mg in 0.1 mL – this can be repeated at 2- to 5-day intervals

one or both eyes and examination of the eye will be quiet anteriorly and posteriorly though there will be patches of white necrotic retina plainly visible. Interestingly while the virus in ARN primarily spreads circumferentially first, in PORN the macula may be primarily involved. Another key difference is that the patches of involved retina in PORN tend to start as multiple areas of small involvement that rapidly spread and coalesce to involve the entire retina (Figure 5.2). This might be compared to civil disorder breaking out all over a country due to the collapse of the state security forces of an unpopular government and within a day or two the protests have involved the entire nation. ARN on the other hand is more akin to the Syrian civil war, in which there are front lines and fighting, in that it fills the eye with inflammation. A diagnosis of PORN usually implies HIV/AIDS if there is no other pre-existing reason found for being immunosuppressed and this must be tested for and HIV specialists involved immediately. From an ophthalmic perspective the prognosis is terrible but every effort should be made to save the affected eye as well as the other if the infection is not yet bilateral. Treatment with oral valaciclovir as in Table 5.8, along with bilateral injections of intravitreal foscarnet repeated at 48-hour intervals can be tried, which may even be combined with oral valganciclovir as well, until the highly active anti-retroviral therapy (HAART) for HIV has worked its best and while the results are still very poor the patient and ophthalmologist can feel satisfied that something at least was done.

CMV retinitis is also a condition which is intricately bound to HIV/AIDS but again other causes of immunosuppression may be at fault. Around half of the adult population has had some exposure to CMV but the immunosuppression results in an opportunistic infection of the retina. Due to the lack of inflammation there is no pain present and as with PORN there is blurred vision and field loss but due to its typically slow nature there are floaters as well. CMV is said to be a 'lazy virus' in that posterior progress is slow but the degree of destruction is great with much intraretinal haemorrhage to the extent that the retinal appearance is often

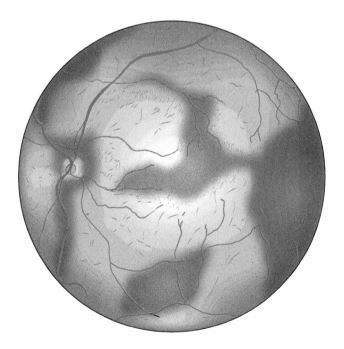

Figure 5.2 Funduscopic view of a patient with progressive outer retinal necrosis.

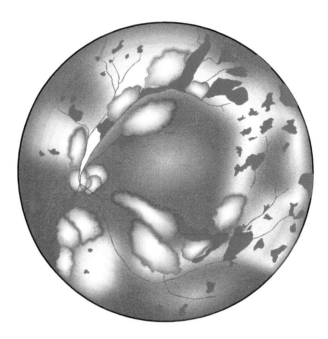

Figure 5.3 Funduscopic view of a patient with CMV retinitis.

compared to a 'margherita pizza' appearance where the exudate, necrosis and blood resemble the melted cheese and tomato of that iconic pizza (Figure 5.3). This starts in the mid-periphery and as with ARN tends to spread circumferentially rather than peripherally. In some patients the retinitis appears as large patches of whitened retina which tend to follow an arcuate pattern along the retinal nerve fibre layer, though without haemorrhage.

As with PORN the main treatment implication is systemic as CMV retinitis is an AIDS-defining illness. An HIV test should be performed, and if positive then an HIV specialist should be involved. With HIV-related diseases the CD4 count is usually very low (<50) but sometimes can be in the region of 50–100. CMV is rare above 100. The retinal prognosis is much more favourable than with PORN and treatment with oral valganciclovir 900 mg twice daily (bd) for 3 weeks followed by 900 mg once daily (od) until the HIV specialist informs you that the immune system is recovered enough for it to be discontinued. As a rule of thumb treatment can be stopped in a patient taking anti-retrovirals if the CD4 has been documented to be above 100 for a minimum of 3 months. An alternative is intravenous ganciclovir 5 mg/kg bd for 2 weeks followed by 5 mg/kg od until the immune system has recovered. Intravitreal foscarnet can also be employed as above but after the first injection the need is not as acute due to the slow spreading nature of the CMV virus. It is useful to take pictures of the fundus with a wide-field camera in this condition as there may be continuing spread of the affected areas that may otherwise go undetected, possibly as a result of patient non-compliance with HAART or virus resistance.

INFECTIOUS ENDOPHTHALMITIS

This subject will be covered in detail in Chapter 6. For now, in the consideration of causes for posterior uveitis, it is of course vitally important to bear this diagnosis in mind in two principal scenarios. First, a patient who has had a recent ophthalmic surgical procedure undertaken such as a cataract extraction and lens implant or an intravitreal injection who then presents with a posterior uveitis with dense vitritis for the first time must be presumed to have infectious endophthalmitis until proven otherwise. Secondly a patient with an acute focus of infection elsewhere such as an infected joint or an abscess associated with septicaemia who suddenly presents with a posterior uveitis is again presumed to have infectious endophthalmitis until proven otherwise. The eye is an ideal organ for growing bacteria; indeed the very reason that vaccinations were previously called 'inoculations' is that the cow eye was used as a perfect culture medium in early microbiology for growing bacteria. Indeed the modern term 'vaccination' is also derived from the Latin word for cow, 'vacca', although that is more to do with the use of the cowpox virus as a primitive vaccination for the much more deadly smallpox virus. The fact that the eye is an immune privileged area under normal circumstances, in which the blood-retina barrier keeps both pathogens and the immune system out, is why any infection can be so quickly devastating. An infectious posterior uveitis, in which bacteria have entered the vitreous through iatrogenic means or through blood-borne spread in a septicaemic patient, very quickly turns into a panuveitis in which no retinal details are visible. In such a patient therefore prompt action is vital and Chapter 6 will tell the ophthalmologist in detail what to do. This includes the rarer infectious causes such as fungal endophthalmitis.

HIGH-RISK TOXOPLASMOSIS LESIONS

Toxoplasma chorioretinitis can cause a severe posterior uveitis which in some cases can be sight threatening. In fact toxoplasmosis is one of the most common causes of a panuveitis in the world. *Toxoplasma gondii* is an intracellular protozoan and the most common cause of human intraocular infection. The natural life cycle of toxoplasma occurs when oocysts get excreted in the faeces of cats which then in turn infects animals such as rodents that would be ordinarily eaten by cats. Inside the intestine of the rodent, termed 'intermediate hosts', the oocyst releases sporozoites after having the tough outer wall broken down by gut enzymes. These sporozoites infect surrounding intestinal cells where they convert to 'tachyzoites' which then go on a colonisation spree all around the host body, though the heart, brain, muscle and retina seem to be preferred places where they settle. Tissue cysts are formed as the immune system besieges these settlements and the tachyzoites transform again into much less active bradyzoites, though occasionally test the defences surrounding them by transforming into tachyzoites in a bid to set up new tissue cysts elsewhere. Cats then kill and eat these rodents and in the feline stomach the tissue cysts burst releasing the bradyzoites which then undergo sexual reproduction forming gametocytes which go on to form oocysts which are released in the gut for the cycle to continue.

The cat must eat the intermediate hosts for the cycle to continue, but unfortunately any land mammal that accidentally comes into contact with the oocysts in cat litter can get infected whether a cat is ever able to eat it or not. There is a large range of animals such as sheep, pigs, birds and humans that if exposed to toxoplasma oocytes in cat litter get infected in exactly the same way as the rodents above. We humans in fact are most commonly infected though not through this method, although children in particular are at risk of eating infected dirt, but through the same way the cats get infected – by eating the intermediate hosts. If all meat is cooked thoroughly and proper hygienic food preparation methods are adhered to no infection should ensue, which is why toxoplasma infection is much more of an issue in the developing world now rather than the West. Contamination of drinking water is also an increasingly recognised source of toxoplasma infection. Unlike in cats the toxoplasma organism cannot sexually reproduce in humans so the consumed tissue cyst containing bradyzoites simply ruptures, the bradyzoites turn into tachyzoites and fresh tissue cysts in the unlucky consumer are then established. The third and final way a human can get infected is if a pregnant woman is herself infected and circulating tachyzoites can then cross the placenta. The chances of this occurring are much greater towards the end of the pregnancy although the clinical manifestation in the foetus is inversely serious. Consequently early infection, while much rarer, can cause the foetus to miscarry. One in 200 live births in the United Kingdom is born already infected with toxoplasmosis. It really is a huge public health issue.

Toxoplasma forms tissue cysts in the retina and if they rupture, releasing tachyzoites, then toxoplasmosis is said to occur. Symptoms of ocular toxoplasmosis are mainly due to the vitritis produced and therefore include **blurred vision and floaters**. Other symptoms such as **photophobia** and **discomfort** are caused by the accompanying anterior uveitis. Optic nerve swelling can be seen either as a result of direct involvement of the juxtapapillary retina or secondary to inflammation elsewhere. Very rarely primary optic nerve involvement can occur in the absence of retinal involvement. The key to understanding the ocular manifestations of toxoplasmosis is this: all the eye features relate to the inflammatory host response to the organism, and this typically occurs both in locality of the lesion – near the retinitis, and more importantly widespread throughout the eye. The degree of inflammation generated can vary enormously from relatively little to a panuveitis. The hallmark finding will be a fluffy white patch of retina, but as explained above, the clinical phenotype is huge. For example, the area of retinitis may be tiny, or very large, or multifocal. If a recurrent infection the new area of activation tends to occur at one edge of the new scar (Figure 5.4), but a scar may not be present, and will not be present at all in primary toxoplasmosis. Vitritis will be present, and typically more evident adjacent to the area of retinitis. In such cases it will look like the classic 'headlamp in the fog' when examined. Severe vitritis can occur, to the extent that no fundal details are discernible, in which case the patient admitting to a history of previous flare-ups of toxoplasmosis can make a big difference

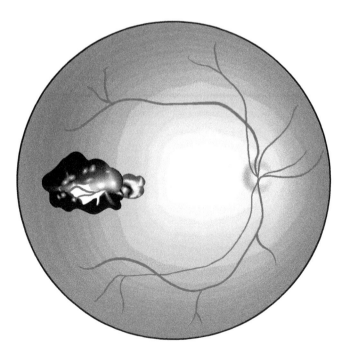

Figure 5.4 A patch of reactivated toxoplasmosis on the border of an old scar with moderate vitritis.

Table 5.9 High-risk toxoplasmosis lesions that require treatment

High-risk toxoplasmosis lesions
Dense vitritis
Lesion located at or adjacent to the fovea or papillomacular bundle
Lesion located adjacent to the optic disc
Lesion located at or adjacent to major arcade vessel
Patient is immunocompromised or immunosuppressed

in guiding management. Retinal vasculitis is common, both venous and arteriolar, and can occur in the locality of the retinitis or be widespread throughout the retina. Segmental yellow-white bead-like plaques can sometimes be seen in the arterioles, called Kyrieleis plaques. If these are present it is highly suggestive of toxoplasmosis.

The greater the posterior inflammation, the greater is the degree of anterior uveitis present, with a **raised intraocular pressure** being a hallmark feature of significant ocular toxoplasmosis. If the patient is immunosuppressed in any way then the degree of inflammation tends to be consequently that much worse.

The diagnosis, as with ARN, is almost entirely clinical. If there is some doubt then blood tests to look for anti-toxoplasma IgG and IgM can be performed. IgG is classically said to be positive if the patient has had previous exposure (the infection is 'Gone') and IgM is positive if the first exposure was recent (the infection is there at the 'Moment'). In practice it is only useful if they are both negative as this would make a diagnosis of toxoplasmosis unlikely but otherwise it is unwise to make clinical decisions based on positive results. If there is some doubt as to whether toxoplasmosis is present or not due to the severity of the disease follow the suggested protocol in Chapter 6. Examination of the fellow eye might be useful in such cases as 40% of cases have toxoplasmosis scars in the contralateral eye.

The next question to ask is whether the toxoplasmosis infection falls into the 'high-risk' category that needs treatment or not. Table 5.9 illustrates what constitutes high-risk disease. If the disease does not fall into this category it is not sight threatening and can be monitored in clinic with a single follow-up appointment in 4–6 weeks to ensure all has settled.

If the disease is sight threatening then treatment should be started immediately. Table 5.10 describes the various treatments available.

The treatment of toxoplasmosis is controversial and various uveitis specialists would put the treatments below in an entirely different order. There is no evidence that any one agent is better than the other. There is weak evidence that the addition of pyrimethamine reduces the size of the eventual scar; theoretically it works synergistically with the others as it has an anti-metabolite action. If you decide to use it get a baseline FBC and repeat every week as it can cause anaemia, low white cell count and low platelets.

LOCAL THERAPIES

If severe disease is poorly responsive to systemic therapy, for example in an immunosuppressed patient, or when for any reason systemic therapy is refused or is contraindicated (see Table 5.10), you can treat toxoplasmosis locally with intravitreal clindamycin 1 mg in 0.1 mL. This can be combined with 400 micrograms intravitreal dexamethasone which can treat the accompanying inflammation. This can be repeated every 1–2 weeks until the disease responds.

If Pyrimethamine is employed then a baseline FBC repeated after a week is needed to check white cells, haemoglobin and platelets. If significant anterior uveitis is also present then topical

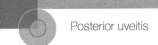

Table 5.10 Treatment of high-risk toxoplasmosis

First line	Azithromycin 500 mg od for 3 weeks.
	In severe disease consider adding: Pyrimethamine 25 mg bd and folinic acid 15 mg three times a week for 3 weeks
Second line	Septrin (co-trimoxazole) 960 mg bd for 3 weeks
	In severe disease consider adding: Pyrimethamine 25 mg bd and folinic acid 15 mg three times a week for 3 weeks
Third line	Sulphadiazine 1 g four times a day (qds)
	In severe disease consider adding: Pyrimethamine 25 mg bd and folinic acid 15 mg three times a week for 3 weeks
Fourth line	Clindamycin 300 mg qds for 3 weeks
	In severe disease consider adding: Pyrimethamine 25 mg bd and folinic acid 15 mg three times a week for 3 weeks
If pregnant	Spiramycin 500 mg qds for 3 weeks
In addition to above, unless immuno- suppressed	Prednisolone 60 mg od 1 week, 40 mg od 1 week, 30 mg od 1 week, 20 mg od 1 week, 10 mg od 1 week then stop Omeprazole 20 mg for 6 weeks

therapy as detailed in Chapter 3 should also be employed. Follow-up in high-risk cases should be in a week to check on progress and to check blood test results if relevant. Once toxoplasma lesions located in high-risk regions, such as juxtafoveally, have settled the thorny issue of prophylaxis needs to be considered. Septrin 960 mg od every other day reduces the chance and severity of a flare-up but as soon as it is stopped the risk returns to normal again. The patient should be made aware of this risk of a flare-up regardless of their taking prophylaxis, and as in high-risk lesions the faster treatment is instituted the better.

If a patient is pregnant and suffers a flare-up of ocular toxoplasmosis the expectant mother can be reassured that there is absolutely no risk to the foetus of infection and spiramycin need only be started if the mother has a sight-threatening infection. This should only be done with the proviso that while the infection poses no risk to the foetus, the treatment does have theoretical risks of teratogenicity. These risks can be avoided by treating locally with intravitreal clindamycin and dexamethasone which is also an option. If the mother suffers primary toxoplasma infection while pregnant then there is indeed a risk to the foetus but in this instance the infectious disease specialist in liaison with the obstetricians should be guiding therapy.

WHAT ELSE COULD BE THE CAUSE OF THE POSTERIOR UVEITIS? ARE THERE DOTS OR SPOTS ALL OVER THE FUNDUS?

All patients reaching this part of our posterior uveitis algorithm by definition do not have one of the three diagnoses described above. The second question to ask is whether dots or spots are present and if so we have a list of differential diagnoses to consider, as described in Table 5.3. The nature of the lesions is paramount in breaking this down; are the dots more like obvious scars with pigment or are they more subtle with less or no pigment? By and large the eyes in which the lesions are more numerous and more obvious are the ones with the greatest degree of inflammation. Although it is a spectrum of dots rather than specific categories, Table 5.11 makes some efforts to differentiate between obvious and less obvious spots. We go through each in turn.

Table 5.11 Obvious and less obvious fundal dots and spots and their associated conditions

Obvious dots/spots	Less obvious dots/spots
Multifocal choroiditis with panuveitis	Presumed ocular histoplasmosis syndrome
Punctate inner choroidopathy	Birdshot chorioretinopathy
Acute posterior multifocal placoid pigment epitheliopathy	Multiple evanescent white dot syndrome
	Sarcoidosis

MULTIFOCAL CHOROIDITIS WITH PANUVEITIS AND PUNCTATE INNER CHOROIDOPATHY

These two conditions will be taken together due to similarities between the two. Indeed some authors have suggested they are a spectrum of the same condition. Multifocal choroiditis with panuveitis (MCP) presents, as the name suggests, with panuveitis which by definition means that the anterior uveal tract is involved, as well as there being obvious vitritis present. The dots or spots are very easy to spot and are usually a mix of older pigmented scars and newer fluffier whiter lesions less than a disc diameter across and usually located in the fundus outside of macula (Figure 5.5). It is said to be a bilateral condition but not infrequently patients do present with unilateral involvement. A hallmark of this condition is the peripapillary presence of lesions which may also be associated with optic disc swelling.

PIC is best thought of as a mild posterior version of MCP. The lesions are still very obvious, unmissable in fact, but are a little smaller at less than half a disc diameter across and located at the macula (Figure 5.6). If each lesion in these two conditions is thought to cause inflammation, the lack of inflammation in PIC versus the panuveitis in MCP can be explained by the

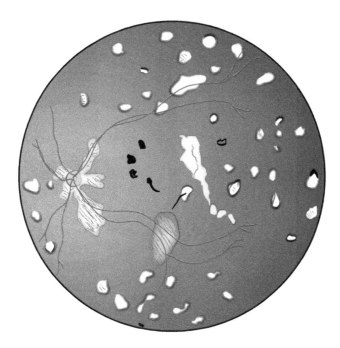

Figure 5.5 Multifocal choroiditis with panuveitis.

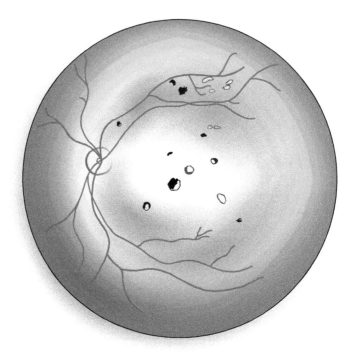

Figure 5.6 Punctate inner choroidopathy.

pure number and area of involvement of these lesions. Again this is said to be bilateral but the patient can commonly present with unilateral involvement. There are conditions that fall somewhere in the middle between these two and although it may be interesting to postulate in an academic (indeed ornithological) fashion which it is, there is no real need to do so. Both these conditions tend to occur in young myopic females.

Both these diagnoses are clinical and no investigations are needed to confirm them or rule out differential diagnoses, though it is always wise to have a low threshold for performing a syphilis serology test. There are two main aims *treatment*-wise: to quieten any inflammation and to treat any choroidal neovascular membranes that may develop. MCP is by definition an inflammatory disorder so treating the anterior segment with topical steroids and cyclopentolate as per Chapter 3, and posterior segment with oral immunosuppression is the usual strategy. The anterior uveitis element usually settles quite quickly if systemic medication is also started and the course of topical therapy needed rarely exceeds 6–8 weeks. Initial immunosuppression is with oral prednisolone 60 mg od for a week, 40 mg for a week, 30 mg for a week, 20 mg for a week, 15 mg for a week then 10 mg for a week. The patient should be monitored during this time and should the inflammation flare up the steroids increased again. Further information on immunosuppression strategy is covered in Chapter 8. The aim of immunosuppression is to treat and prevent CMO and the development of new lesions and scars on the fundus. Serial wide-field fundal pictures are helpful in follow-up to document any changes as the number of lesions means the most artistic ophthalmologist in the world would struggle to document the size, shape and number of them all accurately. Trying to wean the patient off medication is the aim though if repeated flare-ups become a problem a steroid-sparing agent may need to be employed.

In most cases, the active PIC lesions involute to form a scar. In a minority of lesions, the PIC lesions can stimulate the formation of choroidal neovascular membranes as a complication. If these are outside the macula, then conservative therapy is often appropriate as they are not sight threatening. PIC lesions involving the macula are always worrying because of their potential to impair vision for two reasons. Firstly, when they involute into a scar they result in local photoreceptor loss, with resultant central focal scotomas. Secondly, they have a propensity for stimulating secondary sight-threatening macular choroidal neo-vascular membranes.

If a patient presents with a new active PIC-type lesion at the macula an **FFA** is essential to see whether the worsening vision and possible fluid at the macula are due to either inflammation or a choroidal neovascular membrane (CNVM). In the case of the former the angiogram demonstrates a vague ill-defined blur at the affected inflammatory edge of the scar while in the case of the latter the type two membrane that can develop classically lights up early and brightly. The distinction is important as the amount of inflammation produced in PIC during a flare-up is usually very mild if present at all. If a CNVM is the cause of the deterioration then an intravitreal anti-vascular endothelial growth factor (VEGF) injection followed by a review in 4 weeks is the order of the day while if inflammation is the cause an oral course of steroids starting at 60 mg of prednisolone is the recommended treatment with a tapering regime as above. The role of steroid and steroid-sparing agents in PIC is less well appreciated than in MCP and long-term therapy is very unusual. If a clinician is in doubt as to whether an inflammatory flare-up of PIC or a choroidal CNVM is the cause then it is theoretically possible to use both treatments, as they are not contraindicated, although such polypharmacy is usually best avoided as if the patient improves it would not be obvious which of the treatments was effective and thus which needs to be repeated should the patient relapse. It is better to go with the most likely diagnosis initially. If in doubt, you can always review the patient after an interval of 2 weeks with a repeat FFA (or OCT angiography if available). Have a low threshold for changing tack depending on the clinical situation and the results of your investigations.

ACUTE POSTERIOR MULTIFOCAL PLACOID PIGMENT EPITHELIOPATHY

This condition, commonly called APMPPE with the first 'P' being silent, also represents a spectrum of disease though there are a few features that need to be present for this condition to be diagnosed, with the clue being the name itself. Patients are almost always young. It needs to be acute, affect the posterior pole and have multiple lesions present that are placoid, meaning 'shaped like a plate'. This 'plate like' description is best appreciated if you think of an upturned plate as being large, round and slightly raised in the middle with a lower rim around the outside. The fundal lesions look creamy white though after a week can start to become pigmented, hence the 'pigment' in the name. Usually the lesions are around a disc diameter across with the lower edges being slightly fluffy (Figure 5.7) and although the condition is meant to be bilateral there can be significant asymmetry with one eye developing the condition a week before the other in some cases.

Once these basic features are present this condition can be diagnosed although the spectrum varies widely. On the mildest side there are a few placoid lesions present with associated symptoms of blur and visual loss with mild vitritis and no anterior uveitis. On the more severe end of the spectrum there are very many lesions present that can coalesce resulting in a marked vitritis and mild anterior uveitis as well, although the posterior pole should always be visible. Macular involvement can result in permanent injury to vision. In a third of patients there is systemic involvement with all kinds of possible bodily symptoms including a flu-like illness,

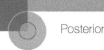

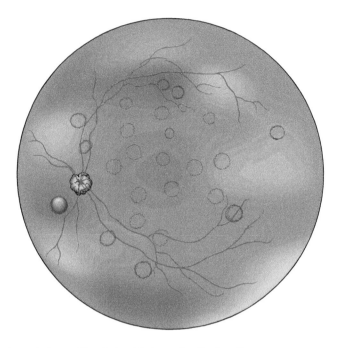

Figure 5.7 Acute posterior multifocal placoid pigment epitheliopathy.

respiratory difficulties, tinnitus, rashes and lymphadenopathy. The symptom to worry about is **headache** as this represents a **cerebral vasculitis until proven otherwise** and if a patient presenting with headache is found to have large placoid creamy white fundal lesions with intra-ocular inflammation then an immediate referral to the physicians for intravenous steroids, usually in the form of methylprednisolone, is mandatory.

Tip: APMPPE can be a life-threatening illness and should a patient be systemically unwell with a headache contact your physicians.

In APMPPE the natural history is for the lesions to self-resolve, ending up as pigmented scars. In many cases the eye is entirely quiet within 3 months. In a minority, the disease becomes chronic, with new lesions continuing to develop. We have come to recognise that this condition can result in severe visual loss, especially if there is macular involvement. Extensive macular involvement, even if acuity is preserved, can result in poor vision arising from para-central scotomas once the lesions involute. The treatment is somewhat controversial as the key decision to be made is whether it is needed at all. The main consideration, for the duration of the inflammation, is whether permanent visual damage to the extent that justifies intervention is likely to take place or not. This would depend on how close the lesions are to the fovea, the disc, and the amount of inflammation present. If a drunk man was slowly stumbling along the road past your house waving a big stick around, the likelihood of you intervening would probably depend on how close he was to your parked car and your property and how aggressively he was waving the stick. Throughout this though, you would question how effectively you would be able to deal with such a situation and would worry about making things worse.

Although the diagnosis of APMPPE is entirely clinical, with large lesions being the hallmark along with an acute history, there are conditions that mimic it and so unlike MCP and

PIC some investigations need to be undertaken. There are many new acronyms for conditions resembling APMPPE but which are due to some other pathology and these change year on year as uveitis specialists attempt to make a name for themselves by trying to classify subgroups of patients into new disease entities. Only the main differential diagnoses need be considered here and even these can be broken down into tuberculosis (TB) and syphilis with regards to investigations. Therefore as a basic rule perform **syphilis serology, QuantiFERON-TB Gold for TB and a chest x-ray**.

The most common differential is the confusingly named **ampiginous** chorioretinitis, which is a variant of serpiginous choroiditis (see below) which as the name implies looks like APMPPE. The rule with serpiginous is that it is caused by TB until proven otherwise, so that rule also applies to this variant that resembles APMPPE. Rather than picking or choosing who to investigate it is better to perform QuantiFERON-TB Gold and a chest X-ray in all cases of suspected APMPPE, although it may be argued that APMPPE is predominantly a disease affecting Caucasians and TB is rare in this group but the rule should still stand for surprises are not uncommon. If your eye department serves a population with high endemic rates of TB such as East London the likelihood of finding a positive association is much greater. A variant of syphilitic eye disease resembling APMPPE is **acute syphilitic posterior placoid chorioretinitis** (ASPPC) which is why a syphilis test should be done routinely in this group. Although ASPPC is said to have fewer and larger lesions in practice it is difficult to tell the two groups apart clinically. Last, though we have mentioned that APMPPE is a self-limiting condition, this is not guaranteed, and an unfortunate minority develop chronic progressive disease termed **relentless placoid chorioretinitis**. For obvious reasons this is a diagnosis that can only be made in hindsight so clinical imaging is key. All other associated conditions will be left to more detailed textbooks to cover as in practice there is nothing that is clinically done differently to the above.

FFA and indocyanine green angiography (ICGA) are not required for diagnosis although the findings are characteristic, with early hypofluorescence and late hyperfluorescence of the lesions demonstrated with FFA, while with ICG there is hypofluorescence over the lesions, suggesting that this is a disorder of the choriocapillaris. Treatment, if deemed necessary by macular involvement or severity of inflammation, is with oral prednisolone 60 mg od for a week, 40 mg for a week, 30 mg for a week, 20 mg for a week, 15 mg for a week then 10 mg for a week. If treated the patient should be followed up initially after a week and then if the condition is improving in two to three weekly intervals until the condition has resolved. If the patient is not on treatment they can be followed up in 6 weeks provided they can be trusted to report any acute visual deterioration which may represent foveal involvement. In most patients, APMPPE will be an acute event that will resolve, with or without oral prednisolone therapy. Sadly the course is not always so benign, and a small but significant minority of patients end up with chronic progressive disease, that will require long-term systemic therapy with steroids and immunosuppression.

PRESUMED OCULAR HISTOPLASMOSIS SYNDROME

This syndrome is one of the many little understood corners of uveitis where the pathophysiology does not really make sense but as nobody knows what is truly going on they are prepared to leave it untouched for now. It is presumed to be due to a fungus called *Histoplasma capsulatum* although the same condition occurs in places far removed from endemic areas and bizarrely having intraocular inflammation, which occurs in true histoplasmosis cases, rules out a diagnosis of POHS. The ocular lesions in this condition exactly resemble those seen in MCP and are all smaller than a disc diameter, usually a third of the size or less, pigmented and arranged classically in lines in the mid-periphery. These spots are termed 'histo spots' and only cause trouble if they are located close to the macula as choroidal neovascularisation (CNV) may develop, which is said to occur in 4% of patients over time.

The classical triad of this condition consists of histo spots, CNV and peripapillary atrophy (Figure 5.8). There almost by definition will be no intraocular inflammation present and if significant vitritis is apparent along with anterior uveitis this condition is called MCP and treated likewise. In fact it is not unknown for people with diagnoses of POHS to flare up and then be reclassified as MCP, so perhaps a better definition of POHS is as a subset of MCP in which the eye has never been documented as being actively inflamed and in which the dots for whatever reason are arranged in lines. It is interesting however as it can present bilaterally but then become apparent in the other eye, all the while without presenting with active inflammation, so it may represent a very benign form of MCP.

The diagnosis is clinical and as with MCP and PIC no investigations are necessary other than an FFA if a CNV is suspected in a macular lesion. If present the CNV can be treated with any anti-VEGF agent though avastin 1.25 mg in 0.05 mL (bevacizumab) is the most commonly used, with follow-up every 4 weeks and treatment on a PRN basis from the outset with no loading phase. Once the lesion has been stable for three visits home monitoring with an Amsler grid can then be instituted. As with PIC lesions if the FFA indicates the lesion may be due to inflammation rather than a CNV immunosuppression in the form of corticosteroids has been known to play a role. The fact that this is true and that antifungals do no good whatsoever is further proof that this is best considered a part of the MCP/PIC family rather than a true fungal infection. As with PIC immunosuppression is with oral prednisolone 60 mg od for a week, 40 mg for a week, 30 mg for a week, 20 mg for a week, 15 mg for a week then 10 mg for a week. Follow-up and OCT scan will determine further action and if all is stable the corticosteroids can be discontinued.

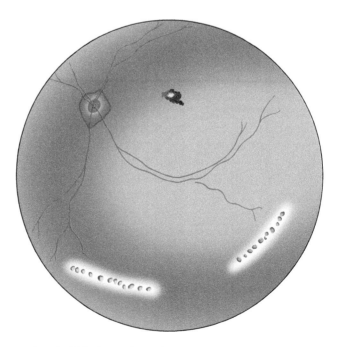

Figure 5.8 Presumed ocular histoplasmosis syndrome.

The vast majority of POHS patients are stable however and rarely need any treatment so home monitoring along with follow-up appointments every year in clinic with fundus photographs is the best way to manage this condition.

BIRDSHOT RETINOCHOROIDOPATHY

Birdshot is a type of lead shot used to kill birds in which the gun discharges multiple small pellets over a wide area which increases the chances of hitting a relatively small moving target such as a bird in flight. This is opposed to buckshot in which larger animals such as deer are hit with a concentrated force of lead which is designed to cause maximum damage in one place as a scattered shot such as birdshot would likely merely annoy a deer which would then run off. It is actually vitally important to understand this before appreciating birdshot chorioretinopathy as the fundus in this condition has bilateral widely distributed lesions that are equally sized and scattered in such a way that it is easy to imagine that they have been shot from a gun. They are almost entirely post-equatorial and spread out more thinly further from the optic disc. They are less obvious than the lesions mentioned in this category thus far as they are cream coloured, not pigmented and around a quarter of a disc diameter in size (Figure 5.9). The view is quite distinctive although the cream colour may be closely related to the natural colour of the fundus and the contrast between the two can make them difficult to see. In this case the green filter on the slit lamp can be very useful to enhance visualisation of the dots.

The typical birdshot patient is a middle-aged Caucasian, usually of North European descent, who presents with blurred vision and floaters as described in Table 5.1 although unlike the other posterior uveitides nyctalopia can also be a problem. The best question to ask here is whether the patient has difficulties in dark environments such as cinemas. The examination is as shown in Figure 5.9 with mild to moderate vitritis and vasculitis being usual but never

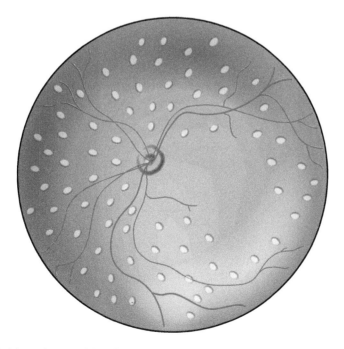

Figure 5.9 Birdshot retinochoroidopathy.

anterior uveitis as birdshot should be regarded as more a smouldering fire than an outright blaze. There are never snowballs or snowbanks present. In line with this the lesions may not be very obvious for years after the onset of the inflammation such that a patient attending with an 'idiopathic' posterior uveitis gradually becomes more obviously a case of birdshot. Both eyes must be affected, but the degree of signs can be highly asymmetrical between the two eyes. In this sense birdshot is quite a sneaky disease and can easily be missed. Intriguingly patients with birdshot occasionally report 'vibrating vision' or a 'wheel turning' in their vision like an old-fashioned fan or a 'shimmering' effect similar to a bright sun glinting on a rolling sea through a seaside hotel window, though these effects are variable and have never been properly investigated. As with most posterior uveitides CMO can be present which can affect central vision while the peripheral effects of the inflammation on the retina can cause visual field changes.

This is a clinical diagnosis and differentials include sarcoidosis, TB, syphilis and intraocular lymphoma, with sarcoidosis the most likely condition to mimic birdshot. The lesions in sarcoidosis (see below) tend to become more pigmented over time while birdshot lesions very rarely do so. The investigations that should be performed include **HLA-A29, FBC, serum angiotensin-converting enzyme (ACE) for sarcoidosis, syphilis serology, QuantiFERON-TB Gold** and a **chest X-ray**. Even though 95% of patients with birdshot retinochoroidopathy are positive for HLA-A29 this should not be regarded as a diagnostic test and its role should be to provide supporting information for the diagnosis. Should there be no characteristic cream lesions present we would not advocate anyone perform HLA-A29 as around 8% of all people in the general population are positive and it may lead to diagnostic confusion. If the test is positive in a person who has the lesions then it carries much more weight.

Angiography also provides supporting information and in this case it is recommended to perform both FFA and ICG. FFA alone demonstrates vasculitis, active leak at the disc (a 'hot disc') and CMO, if present. The lesions are rarely easy to see due to their depth and in practice the fancy descriptions put forward by standard texts do not apply as they cannot be seen. The ICG is very important as the lesions are beautifully highlighted by being hypofluorescent throughout the run. In fact the ICG commonly demonstrates more lesions than the human eye can see during fundoscopy and the marked difference between FFA and ICG is one of the hallmarks of this condition.

The slow-burning nature of birdshot means that neither CMO nor the severity of the vitritis can be used as a benchmark to guide treatment. Of course by following the fundamental principles of uveitis management we must treat both these factors as indications of active disease with increased immunosuppression but even when the eye looks quiet damage can still be occurring. Unusually electrophysiology, in the form of EDT and the ERG in particular, is very useful here. At diagnosis a baseline ERG should be ordered and this often shows markedly reduced *b*-wave amplitude. A 30 Hz flicker delay is also a sensitive and characteristic feature of birdshot, and if CMO is present then the pattern ERG will be attenuated. Once the patient is immunosuppressed the ERG should return to normal unless the patient has chronic damage from long-term untreated disease. Serial visual fields are also useful although they do not replace EDT however, as some patients can show stable electrophysiology with worsening visual fields, a common scenario, and vice versa.

The aim of treatment is to keep the eye quiet and to prevent damage from long-term low-grade inflammation. Oral corticosteroids are initially used although the chronic nature of birdshot retinochoroidopathy means a steroid-sparing agent is almost always needed (Chapter 8). Once the eye is quiet with regard to vitritis and CMO yearly ERGs are used to see if any dose adjustments are needed. Essentially if the ERG *b*-wave amplitude remains normal the dose can be reduced and if this is not the case the dose needs to be increased. It is a mistake to treat the patient with local therapy for observed activity without active monitoring as this 'see-sawing' of inflammation results in a worse long-term visual outcome as well as the accumulated side effects of the local therapy.

Intravitreal steroids may have a role as rescue therapy, with intravitreal triamcinolone, or preferably Ozurdex, used if there is marked CMO in order to achieve temporary control while systemic therapy is initiated. Their short duration of action makes them impractical for long-term use. There is considerable interest in Iluvein, an implant with a longer duration of action. While it appears to control the retinal inflammation, we do not yet know if the implant alone is effective at controlling the choroidal inflammatory driver without systemic therapy.

Tip: **The electroretinogram and visual field play a vital role in monitoring inflammatory activity in patients with birdshot retinochoroidopathy.**

MULTIPLE EVANESCENT WHITE DOT SYNDROME

This is one condition that is very well known but poorly understood. For a start it is probably much more commonly called multiple effervescent white dot syndrome than multiple evanescent white dot syndrome (MEWDS) mainly I would suspect because people never use the term 'evanescent' in daily life and fewer know what it means. Effervescent would imply some kind of fizzy reaction and this is probably why eager eye casualty officers regularly refer cases of MEWDS to the uveitis team when commonly it is APMPPE or MCP present. Another dictum is that an ophthalmologist's first diagnosis of MEWDS is never MEWDS. Evanescent actually means something that quickly fades and disappears, like a snowball in hell perhaps. Patients with MEWDS will almost always be young Caucasian females who present with **blur, para-central scotoma** and **photopsia** classically of one eye but again there are exceptions to this, and in which an initial examination of the eye to the untrained might appear normal. Goodness knows in fact how many MEWDS patients have been passed off as having had a posterior vitreous detachment (PVD) in eye casualties around the world. A common alternative wrong diagnosis is retrobulbar neuritis.

Classically a **prodromal flu-like illness** occurs in the run-up to the eye signs but in reality this only occurs in about 50% of patients. Interestingly the patient may have a striking relative afferent pupillary defect (RAPD), though the patient may already be dilated by the time they make it through to the examination room. A very mild vitritis may be present but the hallmark features are the dots themselves. These are subtle faint white dots at the posterior pole and mid-periphery that are around a tenth of a disc diameter in size. These disappear quickly, as the inclusion of 'evanescent' in the title of the condition implies, although a foveal granularity in which tiny little pixels of orange dots can be seen at the fovea is a sign that lasts a lot longer (Figure 5.10). An OCT scan shows outer retinal changes and if a visual field test is performed due to the patient mentioning scotomas an enlarged blind spot is found on the affected side.

There are no diagnostic blood tests here and there is no treatment to be given. The main differential diagnoses also do not require treatment, so if the history and examination fit there is no real reason to undertake an FFA or ICG. If the dots are missed it might be tempting to label this condition as an acute idiopathic blind spot enlargement (AIBSE) syndrome (see below) or an acute macular neuroretinopathy (AMN – again see below) and the only real way to tell the difference is with angiography, and even then the signs vary. Fluorescein angiography in a MEWDS patient is meant to reveal a 'wreath-like' pattern around the macula in which patchy areas of hyperfluorescence result in a spiky appearance that looks like the Christmas

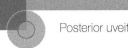

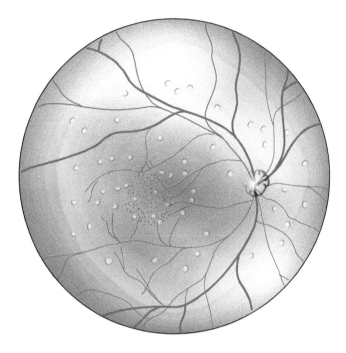

Figure 5.10 Multiple evanescent white dot syndrome.

decoration of the same name hung on doors with the arcades either side and the fovea at the centre (Figure 5.11). In practice this is rare and in fact noteworthy should it occur. The ICG is meant to be much more frequently disordered with hypofluorescent spots corresponding to the white dots. In reality there is no real need to do either of these tests as long as there are no unusual features as it does not change management to do so. There is even less need to perform electrodiagnostic tests so these will not be discussed here.

If a young white patient presents to the eye department with the above symptoms it is always good practice to look for the spots. Without specifically looking for them they will be missed. The main reason for diagnosing MEWDS is not because a treatment exists for it; it is a self-limiting condition that should be gone in 3 months, but to give the patient the right advice and the right prognosis. Confusing a patient with talk of a vitreous detachment and causing worries about their retina falling off, or with retrobulbar neuritis with the associated multiple sclerosis worries, can be avoided if dots are looked for, and if there are no dots but the macula is grainy an OCT and field test, with the rare addition of angiography, can help the treating ophthalmologist give the right advice. A follow-up appointment in 3 months to check all has cleared is prudent, after which the patient can be discharged.

SARCOIDOSIS

This condition has been covered already in Chapters 3 and 4 with regard to its anterior and intermediate mode of presentation. Of interest sarcoidosis is derived from the Greek word 'sarco' which means 'flesh', alluding to the granulomas that form in this condition. While African American, West African and Asian patients have an increased prevalence of sarcoidosis it is not uncommon in the Caucasian population as well with around one in a thousand being

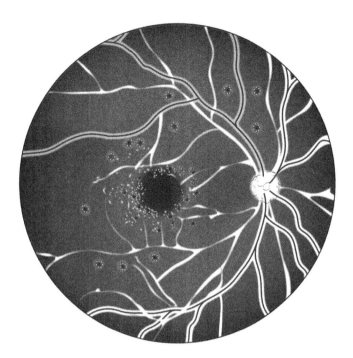

Figure 5.11 The wreath pattern on fluorescein angiography in a patient with MEWDS.

affected. Of the quarter with eye involvement a further quarter of those will have posterior uveitis. Unlike the dots that occur in the conditions listed thus far the dots of sarcoidosis are highly variable and are listed in Table 5.12. The presence of dots or spots in sarcoidosis-based posterior uveitis while useful diagnostically is not at all universal, hence why it is included here in the less obviously seen category.

The spots that resemble multifocal choroiditis are themselves variable but on the whole tend to be less in number, more peripheral and have a predilection for the inferior retina. As in MCP the spots are creamy when active but form a pigmented scar when the inflammation has died down. Occasionally the presentation might mimic birdshot but the presence of pigment in any of the spots should raise the suspicion of sarcoidosis rather than birdshot as by definition birdshot lesions are unpigmented. A patient with posterior uveitis with spots should be asked about **respiratory, joint** and **skin** issues and if any exist a letter sent to the relevant specialty and a chest x-ray organised along with a serum ACE.

If the optic nerve head is involved there is a possibility of neurosarcoidosis, a rare but devastating condition where the sarcoidosis attacks the central nervous system. If a patient who presents to the eye department with suspected sarcoidosis also has a swollen disc and neurological symptoms, even minor ones including a headache, it is advisable to contact the physicians

Table 5.12 Sarcoidosis-related fundal dots and spots

Dot/spot morphology	Cause
Obvious peripheral spots with scarring similar to MCP	Chorioretinitis
One or two large pale raised nodules possibly with subretinal fluid	Choroidal granulomas
Nodular white lesion next to or involving the optic nerve	Optic nerve head granuloma

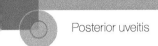

immediately as they will then be able to perform a head computed tomography (CT) scan and lumbar puncture. This is a condition with a definite mortality and morbidity. If there are no neurological symptoms then the swollen disc may be regarded as being potentially due a granuloma rather than disc oedema associated with neurosarcoidosis and a magnetic resonance imaging (MRI) scan as an urgent outpatient can be organised. In the meantime immunosuppression should be started as these lesions can cause dramatic deterioration in vision due to their location. Initial immunosuppression is with oral prednisolone 60 mg od for a week, 40 mg for a week, 30 mg for a week, 20 mg for a week, 15 mg for a week then 10 mg for a week. The patient should be monitored during this time and should the inflammation flare up the steroids increased again. Further information on immunosuppression strategy is covered in Chapter 8.

Many uveitis textbooks talk about the diagnostic criteria for sarcoidosis and how lung biopsies are taken and when thoracic CT scans are ordered but ophthalmologists do not need to know this in any great detail. If there is uveitis, anterior intermediate or posterior, present that looks suspicious of undiagnosed sarcoidosis it is best to ask the patient of any systemic symptoms and if any are present refer the patient to the relevant specialty. Respiratory physicians should organise respiratory tests, rheumatologists examine joints and dermatologists perform skin biopsies. It is advised to order a chest x-ray, a serum ACE and any other test which is indicated if looking for specific other diagnoses but otherwise leave these things alone. Bear in mind that serum ACE is naturally up to 50% higher in children than in adults, for unknown reasons. If the eye condition is suggestive of sarcoidosis and the tests add more evidence but there is no systemic involvement and nothing to biopsy then such patients can be grouped into the 'presumed ocular sarcoid' category, which is an unhelpful dustbin diagnosis that might serve to guide people towards a formal diagnosis in future should systemic signs appear but otherwise adds nothing. If the eye signs are highly suspicious for sarcoidosis consider getting an electrocardiogram (ECG); cardiac involvement can occur in up to 5% and can be fatal. If arrhythmias are detected this may precipitate a referral to the cardiologists.

This section specifically deals with uveitic conditions that have spots and dots but sarcoidosis is better known for the vasculitis it causes, specifically a periphlebitis, although an arteritis can more rarely occur. If this is particularly pronounced ischaemia, neovascularisation and haemorrhage can occur in which case an FFA followed by argon laser to ischaemic areas is called for. Should CMO be present then topical treatment with 6 weeks of Acular (ketorolac) one drop thrice a day is the first step, in addition to treating the posterior uveitis with oral corticosteroids and any anterior uveitis which might be present with a tapering course of topical steroids as detailed in Chapter 3. The treatment strategy for the posterior uveitis is to make the eye quiet then keep it quiet for 2 years. This is initially achieved with a tapering course of corticosteroids and these are then weaned until a safe long-term therapy dose is reached of ideally less than 10 mg of prednisolone a day. If a flare-up occurs then a steroid-sparing agent is started. If the eye remains quiet for 2 years the steroids can then be further tapered until they stop. Chapter 8 has more detail on this.

If there is vasculitis but no dots or spots then sarcoidosis is still a possibility and thus systemic symptoms should be asked about and if suggestive for sarcoidosis the relevant specialties contacted.

IS THERE A VASCULITIS PRESENT?

This question should only be asked at this stage in our diagnostic algorithm once the previous steps have been passed. This is because all significant posterior uveitis is expected to have a greater or lesser degree of vasculitis but in the preceding cases it is not the vasculitis but the presence of other features that points us in the right direction. This section deals with posterior inflammation in which the previous questions have yielded negative answers. Can the type of vasculitis present point us in the right direction? Table 5.4 illustrates some classic associations which help direct our thought processes but there are plenty of exceptions. The first rule of uveitis is that there are no rules. Let's go through each scenario in Table 5.4 in turn.

BRANCH RETINAL VEIN OCCLUSION: BEHÇET'S DISEASE

This condition is named after Hulusi Behçet, a Turkish dermatologist who first described in detail the condition that now bears his name. He worked in a military hospital during the First World War treating soldiers who were fighting the Greek and Allied forces, which may be one reason that in Greece and some Balkan countries this condition is named after Benediktos Adamantiades who was not anywhere near as important as Behçet in describing this condition but was at least Greek. Posterior uveitis in all its forms can cause vasculitis. The hallmark of this is 'sheathing' which as previously discussed is a white layer surrounding a vessel that occurs as a result of inflammatory cells, protein and other material leaking from the vessel itself due to inflammatory mediators breaking down the blood-retina barrier. As it leaks from the vessel it forms a sheath around it in the same way that rust forms around a pipe where the iron is in contact with the oxygen in the air. Simply seeing sheathing is not really helpful diagnostically as it simply indicates an inflammatory process. If there is an associated branch retinal vein occlusion (BRVO) in an eye with posterior uveitis then the first thing to think about is Behçet's disease. This condition affects young adults from the location of the old 'silk road' stretching from Turkey to Japan. In this scenario there are a few specific questions the patient needs to be asked:

Question 1: Where are you or your parents from? Do you have any ancestors from Turkey, the Middle East or central Asia?
Question 2: Have you had any oral or genital ulcers?
Question 3: Have you had any skin rashes, pustules, lumps or bumps?

These are the most important questions to ask. Behçet's disease is a clinical diagnosis and has specific diagnostic criteria based on ulceration and other systemic signs. Again the ophthalmologist does not need to know what the actual criteria consist of as it is the rheumatologist that is best placed to tie everything together. After asking the above questions we can suggest the diagnosis, and refer to physicians who have expertise in diagnosing Behçet's; usually but not always rheumatologists. If the patient denies any systemic symptoms and the above three questions yield negative answers then Behçet's disease is unlikely and referral to a physician at this stage is not advised.

Clinically there are specific features that should alert the clinician to the possibility of Behçet beyond the occurrence of a BRVO with posterior uveitis. Anterior uveitis caused by Behçet classically has a rapid onset and a 'shifting hypopyon'. This is where the hypopyon forms rapidly and as such lacks fibrin so a change in head posture can cause gravity to pull the hypopyon to a new position. While other posterior uveitis conditions tend to cause vitreous cells and debris that coagulate into strings, blobs and other accumulations the lack of fibrin in Behçet causes the whole vitreous to be uniformly 'smoky' with no condensations seen. In addition to the classic BRVO scenario (Figure 5.12) the posterior uveitis can be associated with fluffy white patches on the retina indicative of a retinitis which may be confused with an ARN. Areas of retinitis can commonly affect the macula primarily, which is unusual in ARN (Figure 5.13) – these

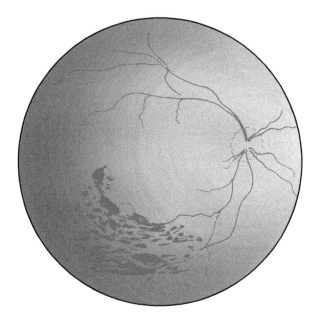

Figure 5.12 Behçet's disease with an associated branch retinal vein occlusion.

infiltrates appear seemingly 'out of nowhere' in terms of their onset and few conditions other than Behçet's disease can do this. In the same way that sarcoidosis can affect the central nervous system in neurosarcoid so Behçet's disease can cause neurological symptoms in a condition called 'neuro-Behçet'. Similarly, though rare, neuro-Behçet can affect the optic nerve. Any neurological symptoms in the context of potential Behçet disease require an immediate referral

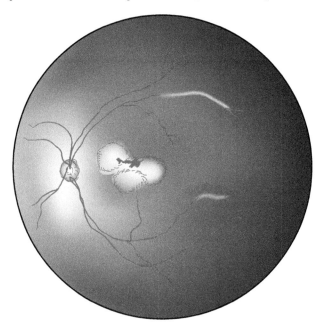

Figure 5.13 Behçet's disease with macular retinitis.

to the physicians who will likely perform an MRI scan of the brain and lumbar puncture to confirm. This is a potentially life-threatening condition and should not be managed in this context by an ophthalmologist.

While Behçet's disease is a clinical diagnosis there are some tests that can be done to provide further evidence, though in reality they are less useful than textbooks suggest. The oft-cited **HLA-B51** test in actual fact is not useful at all and there is no rationale for ordering this except perhaps in some sort of research setting. A patient with active Behçet's disease will often have raised inflammatory markers (ESR and CRP) and also a neutrophilia, but these tests are not diagnostic. You can ask the patient if they report a pustule at the site of phlebotomy. However, the classic **pathergy** test so beloved by textbooks where a sterile needle is used to jab the skin with pustule formation a day afterwards indicating positivity, is unhelpful and should not be done. An MRI of the brain, as mentioned above, should be performed if there are neurological features. If there is evidence of vascular thrombosis then referral to the physicians who can then investigate for other differential diagnoses is best advised. In fact due to the many different specialties which may need to give input to a Behçet patient special combined clinics are set up in some areas to help co-ordinate what would otherwise be a multitude of clinic appointments and a whole rain forest of letters between various doctors. The first step is to ascertain whether your region has such a clinic and if not whether referral to such a clinic in a nearby region would be in the patient's interest.

There are specific diagnostic criteria available for Behçet's disease, much like sarcoidosis above, but as it involves multiple body systems other than the eye it is best a rheumatologist pulls everything together rather than an ophthalmologist. It is better we think of Behçet when faced with a patient with a posterior uveitis who reaches this part of the algorithm, ask questions about systemic symptoms and if the answers are positive refer appropriately. The diagnostic criteria will therefore purposefully not be mentioned here.

It is worth remembering here that TB and syphilis can mimic most uveitic conditions and if the story is atypical of Behçet it is advised to have a low threshold for performing syphilis serology and a QuantiFERON-TB Gold test. An FFA should be considered in all patients with posterior uveitis not so much for diagnostic value but to assess and plan laser treatment for areas of ischaemia. Areas of ischaemia can be much more widespread than clinically apparent and FFA can show extensive capillary non-perfusion. FFA can show a multitude of other abnormalities including vessel staining indicative of vasculitis, arteriolar or venous occlusions and disc leakage.

The treatment of Behçet depends on the overall clinical picture, but it is generally regarded as an aggressive disease which should be treated with shock and awe. If there is anterior uveitis present then this should be treated with intensive topical steroid drops such as Pred Forte at least hourly initially and sometimes half hourly, with a low threshold for subconjunctival Betnesol injection should the uveitis be severe. Cyclopentolate 1% drops for mydriasis three times a day should also be provided. If there is neuro-Behçet present the immediate treatment will be undertaken by the physicians and consists of intravenous pulsed methylprednisolone followed by oral high-dose prednisolone. Due to the aggressive nature of the disease a steroid-sparing agent is usually needed as oral corticosteroids are usually unsatisfactory, with mycophenolate mofetil being a good first choice (Chapter 8) which should be started early.

In the event that ophthalmic manifestations dominate then the form of posterior uveitis present will determine treatment. If vasculitis predominates then oral prednisolone starting at 60 mg and tapering by 10 mg a week until a 20 mg dose is reached is the best treatment, with early commencement of mycophenolate mofetil. If the macula is threatened by a patch of retinitis or vasculitis then intravenous steroids in the form of 1 g methylprednisolone once a day for 3 days followed by oral steroids can be used. An alternative would be to give an intravitreal triamcinolone 4 mg, supplemented with oral prednisolone. Regardless of the strategy, early commencement of mycophenolate mofetil should be considered. Cyclosporin and azathioprine are common alternatives but all clinics seem to treat this condition slightly differently with the only consensus being that its aggressiveness warrants immediate and severe action. Biologics, and in particular, the anti-TNF agents Infliximab and Adalimumab are commonly used in treatment of Behçet's disease, and show good clinical effect (although no randomised control trials exist). They are typically used if there is failure to control the disease despite one or two immunosuppressive agents.

Finally, interferon alpha (IFN-α) has been used for its immunomodulatory effects and has shown benefit in treating both the ocular and the systemic disease in Behçet's. In some cases IFN-α has been shown to produce long-term remission of the disease. Along with flu-like side effects, IFN-α is associated with depression, and all patients must be screened for this prior to and during therapy. This has generally been limited to a few specialist centres.

As with taming a lion, once all these techniques have subdued the condition the dose of oral corticosteroid can be tentatively reduced until it is at or below 10 mg per day of prednisolone and there the treatment should stay until a year has passed, when further reductions can be attempted. If two years of stability are achieved then a plan to discontinue, very gently, the immunosuppression can be instituted but any hint of a flare-up needs immediate and severe action. It is the recurrent severe flare-ups that cause the devastating visual loss in this condition and minimising these is crucial for a good, or at least less bad, outcome. In reality it is rare for a patient with Behçet's disease to be free of immunosuppression, and breakthrough attacks can devastate the vision despite being immunosuppressed so the prognosis is not guaranteed to be good even if correct action is taken. With aggressive modern therapies, including biologics, the visual prognosis is much more favourable than historically, but patients must be aware that this is a potentially devastating disease.

PERIPHLEBITIS: SARCOIDOSIS AND TUBERCULOSIS

Periphlebitis without the presence of a BRVO does not of course rule out Behçet but other diagnoses might be thought of as being more likely. Two conditions stand out for the degree of periphlebitis and sheathing and these are sarcoidosis and tuberculosis. In sarcoidosis the venous exudates caused by the phlebitis can lead to an accumulation of material resembling candle wax surrounding the vessels, a sign called 'candle wax drippings' (Figure 5.14). Tuberculosis is also a possibility and the patient should be asked if they have been exposed to TB or travelled to high-risk areas. If the patient is white and has no history of either exposure or travel then it may be possible to avoid testing for QuantiFERON-TB Gold but otherwise patients with periphlebitis should be investigated with **serum ACE, QuantiFERON-TB Gold, syphilis serology** and **a chest x-ray**. QuantiFERON-TB Gold is discussed below and sarcoidosis has been covered above.

Tuberculosis is one of the most widespread diseases in humanity and has historically affected all civilisations and been responsible for the death of some of history's greatest figures; people such as Franz Kafka, George Orwell and Emily Bronte, not to mention countless monarchs and presidents. TB has myriad effects on every single tissue in the human body besides the lungs and the eyes and patients come to us in two main groups: Those with known TB who have subsequently developed eye problems and those with undiagnosed TB.

The former situation is not really much of a problem. In the common scenario the respiratory physicians would have seen the patient and treated appropriately with antibiotics and asked the

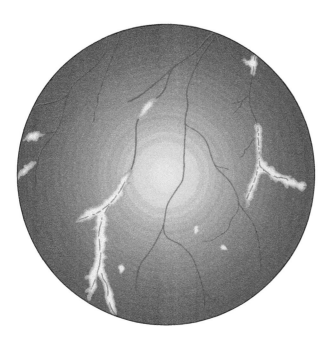

Figure 5.14 Candle wax drippings in a patient with sarcoidosis.

ophthalmologists to see them due to various eye symptoms. The suspicion of ocular TB would be raised and in the vast majority of these patients if any pathology is present it is due to some other condition. This is because the treatment would already have been instituted by the time the patient reaches the eye department and our work is simply to see if anything else is going on.

The alternate scenario, which is far more common, is when a patient turns up with posterior uveitis which our testing reveals to be due to TB. A common third category is where a patient with undiagnosed posterior uveitis has an inappropriate TB test and is sent to the respiratory physicians where after a period of anxiety and delay it is determined that the patient is not to be treated with anti-tuberculous therapy and the real cause can then be looked for. This confusion arises because of the potential for false positives with both of the main investigations, the Mantoux test and the QuantiFERON-TB Gold test. Let us return to the scenario at hand where a patient with a posterior uveitis displaying periphlebitis has entered the clinic. If the patient has obvious vasculitis and a phlebitis in particular then sarcoidosis and TB are the main two conditions to suspect. Look for specific signs of granulomatous disease by re-examining the iris for nodules; examine the corneal endothelium for mutton fat keratic precipitates and scour the peripheral retina looking for whitish dots or nodules that may represent granulomas. Both sarcoidosis and TB can give a similar picture. Also examine the peripheral vasculature for areas of ischaemia caused by vessel obstruction and possible neovascularisation. While these specific vasculitic signs can occur in sarcoidosis, they are more suggestive of tubercular uveitis.

The patient should be asked the following questions:

Question 1: Do you have any breathing difficulties?

Question 2: Do you have any joint or skin problems? Both the above questions apply to sarcoidosis as well which is by far the most common cause of vasculitis in posterior uveitis.

Question 3: Have you been exposed to tuberculosis or visited areas where tuberculosis is prevalent?

If the answer to this latter question is negative and there were no additional features, then the tests to order would include **serum ACE, syphilis serology** and **a chest x-ray**. If the third question was answered positively or there were other supporting features found then you need to start thinking about whether this could be tuberculous uveitis. Unfortunately, at the moment there is no 100% reliable test that can be used to confirm cases of TB-related uveitis. There are however, some common sense principles that at least can be used.

Firstly, consider the likelihood of TB uveitis. This depends on the clinical picture, as well as the local prevalence and the demographics of the patient. For example, TB uveitis is much more likely in an Asian patient who has lived in a TB endemic region, but would be rare in a white patient living in rural northern Europe, or in the mid-Western states of the United States. If TB is a possibility then we need to consider some ancillary testing. We will group these and discuss the usefulness of each in turn:

1. *CXR, CT chest imaging and other more specialist investigations of the chest:* It is reasonable to perform a CXR, but in TB uveitis it is normal in at least 90% of the cases. Furthermore, hunting for TB within the chest with ever more specialist tests such as a CT chest scan, PET scan and lymph node biopsy, or bronchial lavage, is pointless as these are also usually negative and there is nothing to be gained in ordering them. This is no surprise, as in this respect TB uveitis is similar to other extra-pulmonary manifestations of TB such as renal TB.

2. *Gamma interferon assays – the QuantiFERON-TB Gold:* This is said to be positive if the value is greater than 0.35 IU/mL, but in reality it must be interpreted in the context of the overall clinical picture. Limited evidence suggests that strongly positive QuantiFERON-TB Gold values, for example above 2.0, are associated with presumed TB uveitis that responds to anti-TB treatment. Unfortunately, the QuantiFERON-TB Gold has not lived up to initial expectations in terms of its usefulness as a diagnostic test for TB uveitis. For example there is no cut-off value that can accurately discriminate between TB-related and non-TB-related uveitis. More worryingly, the test is not 100% sensitive, and can be falsely negative and the authors have personally seen cases of TB uveitis that have resolved completely with anti-TB therapy, in the presence of a negative QuantiFERON test.

3. *The Mantoux test:* This measures the reaction to intradermally injected tuberculin, and is assessed 2–3 days post injection. It is not a specific test of TB sensitization ('exposure'), as it can be positive with previous bacille Calmette–Guérin (BCG) vaccination, as well as other non-tuberculous mycobacterial exposure. It therefore has high false-positive rates.

Given these drawbacks, it is of less use in assessing TB-related uveitis but on occasions can still be helpful. For example, in a case with clinical features that are highly suggestive of TB uveitis, but with a negative QuantiFERON-TB Gold value, a strongly positive Mantoux would tip the balance in favour of treating with anti-TB therapy. One can also say that a uveitis in the presence of both a negative QuantiFERON-TB Gold and negative Mantoux test is quite unlikely to be TB related. All in all, the field of TB uveitis is therefore very challenging and perplexing for the uveitis specialist. The situation will only improve with the development of novel and more accurate diagnostic techniques that are both sensitive and specific for ocular TB. These are eagerly awaited. Meanwhile, the treatment for TB uveitis is full anti-TB therapy, which should continue for at least 9 months.

The final issue to consider is what to do if the QuantiFERON-TB Gold is positive, but TB is not the cause of the eye condition? What if past exposure to TB caused the positive test result but the inflammation is idiopathic? In this scenario you will need to refer to a chest physician and good communication is essential here. Ultimately you may have to make the call as to whether the eye features could represent TB uveitis or not. If the answer is yes, then you will have to instruct the physicians to commence full anti-TB therapy for treatment of presumed TB-related uveitis, which in all likelihood will be extrapulmonary.

If the eye features are not felt to be likely to be TB-related then this must be communicated to the physicians. They will assess the patient, looking for evidence of latent or active pulmonary disease and treat appropriately. The physicians will also need to know your plans for treatment of the uveitis, as even if the inflammation is not related to TB and the TB infection is latent, giving high doses of systemic steroids, or systemic immunosuppressives, or for that matter biologicals (e.g. anti-TNF agents) can reactivate the bacillus. From the point of view of systemic steroids, the TB mycobacterium is slow at reactivating and there is a 2-week window that exists between starting high-dose corticosteroids and starting antibiotics for treatment of latent TB. Before starting you must be certain of your referral pathway and know for sure that your patient will see the physician and that they in turn know your plan. Good communication is essential here.

The treatment for TB uveitis is anti-TB therapy, which should continue for 9 months. The use of corticosteroids is controversial. If the disease is thought to be inflammatory and the positive QuantiFERON-TB Gold is in turn thought to be due to latent TB then prednisolone 60 mg can be started alongside antibiotics for a week, followed by 40 mg for a week, 30 mg for a week, 20 mg for a week, 15 mg for a week and 10 mg for a week. Further tapering is dependent on the response to the inflammation and if it recurs the dose would need to be increased with slower tapering.

A reasonable question to ask at this stage is whether all people in which high-dose corticosteroid therapy is about to be instituted should be tested for tuberculosis. The short answer is no. The slightly longer answer is that the number of false positives and the sheer weight of numbers of people with latent TB would cause the potential for great harm through mass treatment of people with medications that have very real side effects. The reasonable would then argue that if this is true why treat those in whom we first suspected of having TB which later turned out to be latent with an inflammatory condition being to blame? The answer to this is that if the test is done the result becomes hard to ignore, especially in the rare cases were the bacillus does then become reactivated. Rule number 10 of Samuel Shem's 'House of God' states that if you do not take a temperature you cannot find a fever. This is excellent advice about knowing when not to do tests and of all conditions in this book this is the situation where this most applies.

At this stage it must be mentioned that there is a subset of patients in which ocular TB presents as an occlusive peripheral vasculitis which results in ischaemia beyond the point of obstruction, a condition termed **Eales' disease**. Neovascularisation can then develop. In this scenario as with any neovascularisation following ischemic inflammation laser to the ischaemic area should be undertaken after appropriate mapping with wide-field angiography. While uveitis specialists debate if this particular variant is caused by TB itself, sensitivity to the antigen, or some other mechanism all this discussion is academic to the ophthalmologist faced with a patient with a positive QuantiFERON-TB Gold test and an eye with Eales' disease. The TB needs to be treated with antibiotics through referral to the respiratory physicians and the ischaemic area treated with laser.

BRANCH RETINAL ARTERY OCCLUSION: POLYARTERITIS NODOSA, SUSAC SYNDROME, CAT SCRATCH DISEASE

As with Behçet's disease being associated with BRVO a branch retinal artery occlusion (BRAO) is associated with the above. Association is the important word here as there will always be

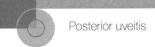
exceptions with other conditions causing an arterial occlusion. All of these conditions are in practice very rare and as with TB the two scenarios will be that either another specialty has made the diagnosis and a referral to ophthalmology was made due to eye symptoms, or that no previous diagnosis was made and we must consider it fresh.

Polyarteritis nodosa, as the name suggests, is an inflammation of arteries and has myriad hideous systemic complications including heart attacks, strokes and infarctions of various organs due to the inflammation of the arteries causing ischaemia. As the eye contains arteries it is possible for these too to become blocked and while embolic branch or central retinal artery occlusion is without any inflammation, should significant inflammation be present it is worth considering this diagnosis. In practice the patient is far more preoccupied by various potentially deadly bodily ills to worry about a missing patch of vision and floaters but there are cases of this being first suggested by an ophthalmologist and should your patient be obviously unwell then immediate treatment with immunosuppression might be lifesaving. Blood investigations will include **FBC, U and E, LFT, CRP, ESR** and **cANCA** as granulomatosis with polyangiitis (GPA) can also very rarely present this way. These investigations are standard investigations for all retinal vasculitides which are not thought to be due to Behçet's disease, sarcoidosis or TB. GPA is the new name for Wegener's granulomatosis, a change which was made due to the fact the Friedrich Wegener was an active follower of the Nazi regime and that at some point he had been wanted by Polish authorities who were investigating war crimes.

Should polyarteritis nodosa be suspected it goes without saying that immediate referral to the physicians is advised and further investigation is best undertaken under them. If the situation is less clear cut then the above investigations can be performed and the patient monitored closely and asked to immediately report any sudden change in condition to the accident and emergency department. From a purely ophthalmic perspective mapping ischaemic areas and treating any neovascularisation with argon laser is the order of the day.

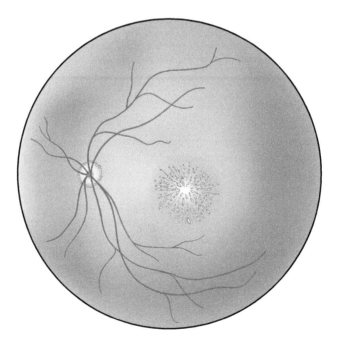

Figure 5.15 Neuroretinitis caused by cat scratch disease.

Susac's syndrome is a triad of branch retinal artery occlusion, hearing loss and encephalopathy caused by a systemic vasculitis affecting arteries. It can be remembered by the phrase 'I'm sorry I can't hear you I have a blinding headache'. As with polyarteritis nodosa it can be potentially lethal and treatment is best undertaken by physicians and immediately so should this be suspected. Again should the situation be less clear cut carrying out the above investigations can help and in this case an MRI scan of the brain can help tip the balance towards Susac and subsequent referral to the physicians. The ophthalmic treatment is related purely to the arteriolar obstruction as detailed above.

Cat scratch disease, caused by a bacterium called *Bartonella henselae,* is a potential cause of vasculitis and branch retinal artery occlusion in particular. It is more widely known for causing neuroretinitis and for this reason it will be dealt with in the relevant section below in detail (Figure 5.15).

ARTERITIS: IDIOPATHIC RETINAL VASCULITIS WITH ANEURYSMS AND NEURORETINITIS (IRVAN)

This book is meant to be a practical guide rather than an in-depth textbook on the intricacies of uveitis. Idiopathic retinal vasculitis with aneurysms and neuroretinitis (IRVAN) is such a rare diagnosis that it will not be considered in depth here except to say that if a vasculitis is present and the arteries are primarily involved then aneurysms should be looked for as in this condition there are multiple macroaneurysms along the arteries, hence the name. Interestingly immunosuppression has no great effect here and the mainstay of treatment is argon laser to obliterate the areas of ischaemia that occur following occlusive arteritis. The rarity of this condition of such that while there is no definitive diagnostic test more common diagnoses that might respond to immunosuppression or other treatment need to be excluded.

SYPHILIS

This great mimicker of almost all other inflammatory eye conditions should always be considered to a greater or lesser extent but its usual manifestation is with posterior uveitis with a vasculitis. Otherwise from the cornea at the very front to the optic nerve at the back syphilis can mimic any condition so if the presentation of another form of uveitis is slightly more unusual than expected always test for it via a syphilis serology blood test. All posterior uveitides where vasculitis is the most prominent feature should have syphilis testing. Syphilitic vitritis may range from mild to so severe that the fundus cannot be seen. Fluffy cream lesions less than a quarter of a disc diameter dotted over what appears to be the surface of the retina would come under the 'unusual' category as it does not fit in with what we have seen thus far. Despite the notorious reputation syphilis has as a mimicker of other conditions, there are a few aspects of ocular syphilis that might alert you to this possibility.

Syphilis is the name given to the clinical condition caused by the spirochete, a spiral-shaped gram-negative bacterium, *Treponema pallidum*. This condition is famously spread through sexual contact and a positive diagnosis can have wide-ranging social sequelae. In the United Kingdom and North America syphilis is the overwhelming preserve of men who have sex with men (MSM) while in China and Africa heterosexual transmission, and prostitution in particular, is much more important. It is not a preserve of the young, so do not forget to test in the elderly, as studies show a broad range. Other than uveitis there are myriad other bodily manifestations of syphilis involving hands, feet, skin, mucous membranes and neural tissue. Remember that syphilis can cause hearing loss and this can also alert you. In practice as ophthalmologists rarely understand skin rashes, do not perform neurological examinations very well and almost never examine external genitalia these signs will not be discussed here as they are simply not useful to us in being able to diagnose the condition. Instead we see that the uveitis is unusual and we ask the patient two identical questions every time:

Question 1: Don't worry we ask these questions of everyone with an inflamed eye like this.
How many sexual partners have you had in the past 6 months?
Question 2: Were they all men, women or both?

These questions are sensitive and must be asked in a confidential environment where the patient is relaxed enough to give as truthful an answer as possible. If there is a friend or relative accompanying the patient it stands to reason that they be asked to sit outside otherwise it becomes pointless asking the questions. In reality, even with the most confidential environment in the world, the complete absence of horrified spouses and with the most sexually relaxed and accepting ophthalmologist in Christendom, the first time these questions are asked the answers are often less than entirely truthful. After asking the questions tell the patient that in with the regular blood testing there will be a test for syphilis as this is 'routine and all patients in this situation have this test'. Never let the answer dissuade you from performing a blood test for syphilis; the purpose of asking them is to let them know you are indeed performing it and every so often truthful answers are given which can result in an early referral to a genitourinary medicine (GUM) clinic. It is not uncommon for patients to get angry in clinic if handed a blood test form with 'syphilis serology' ticked when the above conversation has not taken place.

Syphilis blood testing can be confusing to the ophthalmologist. This should not be the case however as in reality it is really simple. If you tick 'syphilis serology' on the blood test form, then a modern lab in the developed world (Europe and North America) will do either the FTA (fluorescent treponemal antibody absorption test) or syphilis IgG. **Never** use the 'VDRL test' (which stands for venereal disease research laboratory) to test for syphilis and never write this on the form. This test along with the rapid plasma reagin (RPR) are older tests and are not even specific tests for syphilis. They work by detecting antibodies to cardiolipin-lecithin-cholesterol antigen. A number of other conditions falsely react with this – including systemic lupus erythematosus (SLE), Lyme disease and IV drug abuse. More worryingly, these tests can be falsely negative in late syphilis disease.

The FTA and IgG are specific and highly sensitive antibody tests for syphilis, and if positive indicates that the individual has been exposed to *Treponema pallidum* at some point in his or her life. They remain positive forevermore, regardless of whether the patient receives treatment or not. In the context of a patient with active eye inflammation with a positive test the patient must be considered to have syphilitic uveitis until proven otherwise and will need an urgent referral to your genitourinary medicine colleague. This point is so important it will be repeated; use the FTA or syphilis IgG when looking for syphilitic uveitis. The VDRL and RPR are not entirely useless however and can be used to assess how active the infection is. You do not have to worry too much about this as the genitourinary physicians will guide you, but most of your patients with syphilitic uveitis will be in the secondary stage of syphilis, with very high VDRL or RPR titres.

Syphilis is treated by the GUM physicians. It should never be treated by ophthalmologists. There are two interesting features of this organism: Lack of resistance and the Jarisch–Herxheimer reaction. The spirochete itself seems unable to develop a resistance to penicillin, and despite the development of antibodies, humans can be re-infected. Intramuscular benzylpenicillin over a period of between 2 and 3 weeks is the usual treatment, provided of course the patient is not allergic. The genitourinary team will ask the sensitive questions so contact tracing can take place, consider HIV testing and organise the antibiotic treatment itself. The sudden death of huge numbers of organisms following penicillin commencement can result in the Jarisch–Herxheimer reaction where the sudden increase in antigen load can cause a worsening of inflammation around the whole body. This can be managed by concurrent oral steroid administration but for obvious reasons this is a fine balance and so should be controlled by the genitourinary physicians. Our role is to monitor the eyes through this process – administrating topical steroids should anterior uveitis become a problem and advising our GUM colleagues about the steroid dose should the posterior inflammation worsen during treatment.

Finally, a group of similar treponemal bacterial infections called yaws and pinta are present in poor communities in warm, humid, tropical areas of Africa, Asia, Latin American, the Caribbean and the Pacific. These cause skin, bone and cartilage infection. While they can affect the face and eyelids they do not really cause intraocular inflammation and are not sexually transmitted. The problem is that they will result in positive FTA and IgG tests, as they cannot be distinguished from *Treponema pallidum* syphilis. In the United Kingdom you might come across patients who were brought up abroad who will have evidence of yaws, usually with scars on their legs, and as a consequence they will have false-positive *Treponema* serology. What also must be considered is if in such a patient an active eye inflammation is also present there is no reason why they cannot also have a coexisting sexually acquired syphilis infection with *Treponema pallidum* just like anybody else! Previous yaws or pinta infection does not protect against sexually transmitted diseases of any kind. You will have to decide whether the positive blood test is a red herring and you will need a thorough GUM assessment. It is not uncommon in such scenarios to make a pragmatic decision to err on the side of caution and treat such patients with penicillin.

In terms of the ocular findings in syphilis any structure can be involved, though there are a few features that might raise your suspicions. In 50% of cases the inflammation is bilateral but it can be highly asymmetrical. Different structures can be involved in the two eyes, for example a swollen nerve in one eye and a patch of retinitis with vasculitis in the fellow eye, and other than with Lyme disease this feature is most unusual in other uveitic diseases. In unilateral disease the left eye is affected more frequently although the reason for this intriguing fact is not known. Additionally syphilis rarely presents with anterior uveitis in isolation without any intermediate or posterior segment signs whatsoever, though these may be subtle. Distinctive clinical pictures include the following:

1. Small yellow-white round spots of inner retinitis called syphilitic inner punctate retinitis are present.
2. Acute syphilitic posterior placoid chorioretinitis is found (see APMPPE above).
3. Optic neuritis can present as a swollen optic nerve (anterior optic neuritis) or when the optic nerve head appears normal posterior optic neuritis can be detected clinically via loss of visual acuity, impaired colour vision and the presence of an RAPD.

Tip: **Syphilis can mimic any uveitic condition of the eye and there should be a low threshold for testing if it is suspected.**

IS THERE A FUNDAL LESION PRESENT AS PART OF THE POSTERIOR UVEITIS SYNDROME THAT DOES NOT FIT INTO THE ABOVE CATEGORIES?

This last category of posterior uveitides includes those in which there is no immediate sight-threatening lesion, in which spots or dots do not form the dominant feature and in which vasculitis, while possibly present, does not present in a severe or distinctive manner. There are however distinctive lesions present that enable some form of identification and a narrowing of the list of differential diagnoses.

PIGMENTED PATCH OF RETINA WITH WHITE FLUFFY PATCH AT ONE MARGIN: TOXOPLASMOSIS

High-risk toxoplasmosis lesions were covered earlier in the sight-threatening category. These lesions are described in detail in Table 5.9 and are mainly anatomical descriptions of high-risk locations. It is far more common to find the reactivated toxoplasmosis lesion in some mid-peripheral patch of the retina and unless there is significant vitritis present no treatment is usually needed in these cases. Remember that toxoplasmosis-based uveitis is commonly associated with a rise in intraocular pressure. A follow-up in 6 weeks to make sure all is well may be indicated.

PERIPHERAL MASS WITH FIBROGLIAL TRACTION: TOXOCARIASIS

Where toxoplasmosis is a cat-borne disease, toxocariasis is spread by dogs. *Toxocara canis* is a nematode worm that is thought to infect the vast majority of household pups. There is in fact a cat variety called *Toxocara cati* although this is far less important from a human infection perspective. The adult worm lives in the gut of infected dogs happily passing eggs into the faeces which, due to the canine habit of eating faeces, then infects another dog. The eggs after ingestion develop into larvae and pass through the gut wall into the circulation and hence in the blood to the dog's lungs, where they are coughed up and swallowed. These then grow into adult worms and further their own species' existence by passing new eggs into the faeces for other dogs to get infected. Humans are accidental hosts and almost always get infected by coming into contact with dog faeces, either through accidental contamination or the horrible habit some children have of eating soil. For this reason, as well as an increased natural susceptibility, very young children form the biggest group of people with primary *Toxocara canis* infection, although the sequelae last a lifetime. It is for this reason there are signs in parks warning dog owners to take their dogs' faeces home with them because 'dog waste can cause blindness'.

In humans the ingested eggs cannot mature into an adult worm as the larvae travel the body looking for the lungs but due to differences in physiology with dogs get utterly lost and end up in the wrong organ. After their failed journey to find the lungs the larvae either die or get isolated in a covering of inflammatory tissue called a granuloma. The majority of the larvae die at the time of infection and this mass death causes an immune response which in the majority is asymptomatic although in some, almost entirely very young children, a condition called visceral larva migrans can occur. This is a systemic disease of fever and eosinophilia caused by the immune reaction against dead and dying larvae and further symptoms are related to where the larva ended up. If in the brain encephalitis can occur, if in the liver hepatitis and if in the heart myocarditis. As the reaction is due to the death of the larvae anti-helminth drugs have no place here, although steroids may dampen down the reaction. This may be of peripheral interest to ophthalmologists as it will be the paediatricians tasked with treating this potentially life-threatening disease, but it is important we ask about it as the discovery of an ocular granuloma in an older child or adult will very much mean *Toxocara* is something to consider if the patient or their parents recall a time when they were very ill when they were very young.

Eye wise there are three main ways *Toxocara* can present: A diffuse chronic endophthal-mitis, a posterior pole granuloma and a peripheral retinal granuloma, in decreasing order of severity and thus increasing age of presentation. The **chronic endophthalmitis** presents in primary school-age children with a panuveitis the defining feature of which will be signifi-cant macular oedema and bands of gliosis, which can be associated with a tractional retinal detachment. Basically the inside of the eye is inflamed and scarred. This presentation results from a dramatic immune response to larval death. If the larvae survive long enough to form a granuloma proper the eye is protected from inflammation and the larva is protected, to a cer-tain extent, from death. There is less inflammation associated with this variety, hence an older age of presentation, but if the granuloma happens to be at the **posterior pole** the disruption to central vision caused by scarring and tractional bands on the macula will bring it to the atten-tion of parents and healthcare professionals usually before the child leaves secondary school (Figure 5.16). If the granuloma happens to be **peripheral**, which in fact is where most *Toxocara* granuloma are located, the effects to central vision may be limited and presentation may be in adulthood (Figure 5.17). The retinal appearance in the cases of these granulomas is of gliotic masses with tractional vitreous and retinal elements surrounding them that can distort the retina to a greater or lesser degree, and of a vitritis which varies from fulminant to very low grade only affecting the vitreous directly overlying the lesion itself.

The natural course of ocular *Toxocara canis* is to be inflamed from time to time due to immune action against an encapsulated protected invader with the gliotic traction forces becoming more important over time. The main differential diagnosis due to the age and appearance of a nodu-lar mass is retinoblastoma, but although the ages do overlap *Toxocara* tends to present in older children. Toxoplasma is another common differential, though here the mass is flatter rather than nodular and the tractional elements are much less important. The diagnosis is clinical and the question that must always be asked is 'do you have dogs in the house'? A negative answer

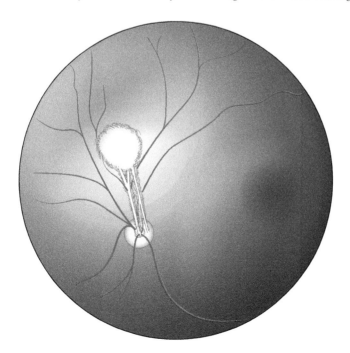

Figure 5.16 A posterior pole retinal granuloma associated with *Toxocara canis* infection.

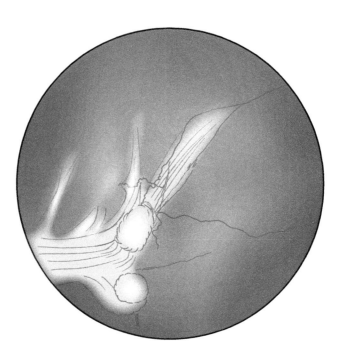

Figure 5.17 A peripheral retinal granuloma associated with *Toxocara canis* infection.

of course does not rule out this diagnosis but a positive one reinforces it. Serology for *Toxocara*, like many other tests in the field of uveitis, have an issue with sensitivity and specificity so, as with the question about dogs, provide more of a guide than an absolute answer. B-scan ultrasound of the eye is a useful diagnostic test as it can differentiate between retinoblastoma and *Toxocara* granuloma, although if there is any doubt here it is better to refer to an ocular oncologist.

As the symptoms come about through inflammation related to larval action the treatment is in the form of periocular steroid and topical steroid for vitritis and anterior uveitis, respectively, with the possibility of systemic steroid related to the weight of the child and in joint care with the paediatricians in the event of significant inflammation. The orbital floor injection may need to be given under sedation in theatre if the child is young although the majority of *Toxocara* cases may not need any treatment at all. If vitreous bands and tractional detachment become an issue then referral to a vitreoretinal surgeon is advised so these forces can be countered, under anti-inflammatory cover of course. Paradoxically drugs that target the worm itself, called anti-helminthics, are actually of no use. This is because they do not penetrate the granuloma and have significant side effects. It could be argued that the inflammation, which is actually what causes the symptoms, is caused by larval death and so killing the organism is likely to make things worse. This is just conjecture however as no evidence exists one way or another. Over time, unless the patient is exposed again and again to more *Toxocara* eggs, the larvae die off and although the vast majority die shortly after infection some have been hypothesised to survive for decades inside granulomas. But nobody really knows.

There are other ocular diseases caused by worms, namely diffuse unilateral subacute neuro-retinitis (DUSN) and onchocerciasis, also called river blindness. These diseases are fascinating and covered in quite a lot of detail in many textbooks but unlike *Toxocara canis* are vanishingly rare in a typical Western ophthalmic practice and will not be considered here. Every time I have myself considered any one of these rare diagnoses it turns out to be an unusual presentation of a far more common disease.

EXUDATIVE RETINAL DETACHMENT WITH OR WITHOUT NODULES OR SPOTS: SYMPATHETIC OPHTHALMIA OR VOGT–KOYANAGI–HARADA SYNDROME

These two conditions are almost identical, with only the history separating them. They are both rare but do occur often enough to warrant more than an academic consideration in diagnosing posterior uveitis. The specific sign that differentiates these conditions is the exudative retinal detachment. Many causes of posterior uveitis, as well as non-uveitic conditions, can cause an exudative detachment, though these two conditions are so famous for it that should a striking exudative detachment be present then these conditions should be considered first. Sympathetic ophthalmia is a condition that occurs in the contralateral eye following trauma or multiple surgeries, which is a form of trauma, to an eye. The damaged eye is known as the exciting eye as the damage is thought to release some as yet unknown antigen into the blood that causes an immune response against it that then goes on to involve the other eye, called the sympathising eye. Perhaps it is easier to imagine twin brothers where one twin gets into trouble with the police who take his picture and then go on to harass the innocent twin purely because of the trouble the first one caused as they look so identical the police cannot tell the difference.

After excessive damage to one eye occurs and visual potential is nil then enucleating the eye within 10 days of the injury is said to reduce the chance of sympathetic ophthalmia occurring. The evidence is scanty however, the visual potential cannot be easily predicted after an injury and the patient may end up with a worse cosmetic and psychological result after an early enucleation so in practice this policy is rarely followed. Once the immune system is sensitised however, once the bad twin is 'on file' so to speak at the police station, there will always be a risk to the good twin for the rest of his life. The file is never destroyed. The history must involve trauma or surgery to one eye with the other eye presenting with panuveitis.

If and when sympathetic ophthalmia does occur, the history of visual deterioration, blur and floaters in the sympathising eye can be sudden over several days or less commonly build slowly over a few weeks. There is anterior chamber inflammation, which is often but not always granulomatous, and examination of the posterior segment can reveal significant and sometimes severe vitritis, with optic disc swelling, macular oedema and the two most important and distinctive features: Small round yellow nodules mostly in the periphery called Dalen-Fuchs nodules and striking areas of serous retinal detachment that look like multiple blisters that may coalesce (Figure 5.18). After treatment over time the Dalen-Fuchs nodules become pigmented scars and the swollen optic disc shrinks into an area of peri-papillary atrophy. Retinal vasculitis is almost never seen, and for practical purposes this can help distinguish it from other causes of panuveitis. The spectrum of disease severity in sympathetic ophthalmia varies widely, ranging from devastatingly severe posterior segment disease to very mild disease and in rare cases a mild anterior uveitis may be the only manifestation.

Vogt–Koyanagi–Harada (VKH) syndrome is best thought of as a form of systemic sympathetic ophthalmia that affects both eyes. While it was traditionally thought of as a disease of East Asian peoples, it is now recognised as occurring in individuals with pigmented skin, of all ethnicities in the world, including the Far East, Africa and South America, though interestingly India arguably has the highest prevalence. It rarely occurs in Caucasians, including White

(a)　　　　　　　　　　　　　　　　　(b)

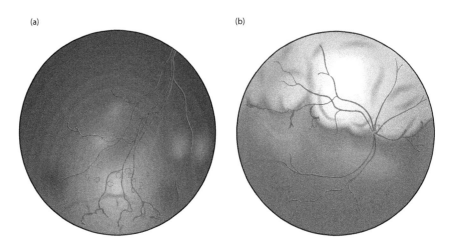

Figure 5.18 Fundal view in sympathetic ophthalmia and Vogt–Koyanagi–Harada syndrome.

Europeans, but it is almost unheard of in people of Northern European ancestry. The fundal appearance is identical to that seen in sympathetic ophthalmia but without the history of trauma. Patients with this condition will present to us in the eye department due to a short history of blur and floaters, similar to sympathetic ophthalmia, though in both eyes. Examination is as in Figure 5.18 with the areas of exudative retinal detachment, optic disc swelling and small round yellow nodules being the distinctive features, but of these the exudative detachment is the most important sign. The distinguishing features, other than the history of trauma, include the likely ethnicity of the patient and the systemic signs.

The systemic disease might be regarded as a racist immune system, in that the melanocytes in pigmented tissues are targeted and destroyed. As with many similar conditions it is hypothesised that some form of virus triggers a susceptible immune system into misbehaving in this way, but nobody really knows. There are melanocytes present in the meninges and inner ear organs such that early signs are of malaise and headache due to meningeal inflammation, sensorineural hearing loss, tinnitus and vertigo. This prodromal stage is followed a few weeks or months later by the acute uveitic stage. A sudden-onset bilateral granulomatous uveitis develops; by definition the disease must be bilateral although a short interval of about 2 weeks can occur in between first and second eye involvement. The typical features, as with sympathetic ophthalmia, are a granulomatous anterior uveitis with mutton fat keratic precipitates and peripheral synechiae. Posterior signs include vitritis, disc hyperaemia, pockets of serous retinal detachments and choroidal lesions. Occasionally, annular serous detachments cause the lens iris diaphragm to move anteriorly and patients can present with an acute secondary angle-closure glaucoma that is not due to pupil block. These patients can mistakenly receive laser iridotomies via the glaucoma team, an entirely pointless intervention as the correct therapy is with steroidal immunosuppression.

As mentioned in Table 5.13 there are specific FFA features of note, namely multiple early focal hyperfluorescent spots with later pooling in areas of serous retinal detachment. In the acute stage enhanced depth OCT imaging is useful as it shows subretinal fluid and a markedly thicker choroid. ICG is very important here as the primary site of pathology is the choroid. Three changes have been described, all three indistinguishable from sympathetic ophthalmia, and these are early hyperfluorescent choroidal vessels, 'fuzzy' or indistinct large choroidal

Table 5.13 Criteria for diagnosing the three variants of Vogt–Koyanagi–Harada syndrome

Criteria	Symptom or sign
1	No history of ocular surgery or trauma
2	No evidence of any other cause for uveitis
3	Bilateral uveitis with
	• If early disease
	• Subretinal fluid
	• If no subretinal fluid characteristic FFA findings with choroidal thickening
	• If late disease
	• History suggestive of the above
	• Sunset glow or Sugiura's sign
	• If no sunset glow or Sugiura's sign: Choroidal scars, RPE pigment clumping and recurrent or chronic anterior uveitis
4	Neurological or auditory symptoms
5	Poliosis, vitiligo or alopecia

vessels and hypofluorescent dark spots. Choroidal thickness is a useful measure if available as it can be used as a surrogate measure of response to therapy, with adequate therapy resulting in normalisation of thickness, though chronic undertreated disease can result in the choroid becoming abnormally thinned.

A few weeks or months after onset the skin melanocytes can be affected with symptoms of poliosis (whitening of the hair), alopecia and vitiligo. The racial predilection of the patients is such that there are two additional signs that are specific to this condition. Peri-limbal conjunctival pigmentation, known by various names which change due to variances in racial sensitivity over time, is a phenomenon more prevalent in the darker skinned and East Asian races. The current name in vogue seems to be complexion-associated melanosis (CAM). The immune attack launched in VKH can eliminate these natural peri-limbal pigmented patches and this disappearance is known as Sugiura's sign. The fundi of darker-skinned individuals also tend to be browner and less orange than that of a Caucasian and immune attack on the melanocytes contained in the choroid can over time result in a more orange glow than you expect, the 'sunset glow' sign. However, if prompt and appropriately aggressive systemic therapy is started, these late signs are rarely seen these days.

As with sympathetic ophthalmia the Dalen-Fuchs nodules over time form pigmented scars that may resemble multifocal choroiditis, and as with any pigmented retinal scar there is always the possibility that choroidal neovascular membranes can grow through these defects and bleed.

Tip: **Think of VKH if your patient has pigmented skin but remember that it can occur in Caucasians.**

The diagnosis of both conditions is entirely clinical, though in the case of VKH syndrome there are five specific criteria based on the systemic as well as ocular findings which tell you which of the three variants of VKH is present. Table 5.13 gives these criteria, with Table 5.14 showing the variant based on the criteria in Table 5.13.

In practical terms the ocular features of VKH plus headache alone remain probable VKH and were not sufficient for making the diagnosis of incomplete or complete; this phenotype has been called Harada's disease although you should be wary of making this diagnosis. Most patients present to ophthalmologists first and taking a good history that includes asking about

Table 5.14 Naming the form of Vogt–Koyanagi–Harada syndrome present based on Table 5.13

Criteria present	Name
1, 2, 3	Probable VKH (ocular VKH)
1, 2, 3, 4 or 1, 2, 3, 5	Incomplete VKH
1, 2, 3, 4, 5	Complete VKH

hearing problems is key as the symptoms can be easily overlooked. Patients with ocular findings and hearing problems but no other neurology do not need referral to a neurologist; they have little to add in the management, which will essentially be driven by the eye disease. Patients with ocular findings and any other hard neurological signs other than hearing problems, a cranial nerve palsy for example, need immediate referral to neurology for co-management as these patients have serious morbidity and potentially life-threatening disease.

In terms of the differential diagnosis only a relatively small number of diseases can mimic VKH. First, ask about a history of ocular trauma, as this raises the possibility of sympathetic ophthalmia, which is the main differential diagnosis. APMPPE can clinically resemble VKH though an FFA will help you weed out APMPPE as the difference is obvious. It is always necessary to perform **syphilis serology** as syphilis, the great mimicker, has been known to mimic VKH, both with uveitis and hearing problems. Table 5.15 lists conditions in which hearing loss occurs in the presence of uveitis.

It has been known for East Asian patients with what appears to be VKH to suffer significant delayed diagnosis of syphilitic uveitis. Never stereotype. Posterior scleritis must be considered in the differential diagnosis of all VKH patients, as it can present with many similar signs, including disc oedema, subretinal fluid, choroidal lesions and a degree of anterior chamber activity and vitritis. A B-scan ultrasound is key to the diagnosis as it will identify sub-Tenon's fluid, the 'T sign', which will be absent in VKH (see Chapter 7). Rarely sarcoidosis or ocular TB can share some common features but there are always distinguishing features such as the presence of vasculitis, which is not seen in VKH. Finally, uveal effusion syndrome may superficially resemble VKH as it can cause serous retinal detachments, but the absence of inflammation is a major distinguishing feature here.

The treatment of sympathetic ophthalmia and VKH is pretty much the same – immediate high-dose oral steroids. This is combined with intensive topical steroids and cycloplegics to treat the anterior uveitis. In cases of VKH with particularly severe eye inflammation – eyes with massive exudative detachments for example – initial therapy with pulsed intravenous

Table 5.15 Conditions that cause hearing loss in the presence of uveitis

Diseases that cause both hearing loss and uveitis
Vogt–Koyanagi–Harada syndrome – and very rarely sympathetic ophthalmia
Sarcoidosis
Syphilis
Lyme
Relapsing polychondritis – both auricular pain and sensorineural deafness
Granulomatosis with polyangiitis (formally Wegener's disease) – both sensorineural and conductive deafness
Susac's syndrome
TINU – tubulointerstitial nephritis and uveitis

methylprednisolone is preferred in the form of 500 mg of intravenous methylprednisolone once a day for 3 successive days, followed by a tapering regimen of oral prednisolone starting from 60 mg a day. For less severely affected cases the patient can pass immediately to the oral prednisolone stage, generally at either 60 mg or 1 mg/kg per day, initially for 2 weeks with subsequent tapering of the daily dose by 5 mg decrements per week down to 20 mg daily. Thereafter tapering is undertaken more slowly, with 2.5 mg decrements every 4 weeks. The treatment is individualised depending on the response. Steroid treatment must be given for an absolute minimum of 6 months, though the reality is that most patients will require steroid therapy for about 18 months to 2 years. Given the relatively high steroid threshold of this disease, early introduction of steroid-sparing immunosuppressives should be considered. All have been tried, including anti-metabolites and calcineurin channel blockers but the choice ultimately depends upon clinician preference and how quickly you want an effect. While T lymphocytes have an important role in driving the choroidal element of the disease it stands to reason that T-cell inhibitors like cyclosporine or tacrolimus might be preferable, though there is a distinct lack of actual evidence and it is not uncommon to find what is theoretically true at odds with reality in the voodoo cult of uveitis.

Local therapy is potentially useful and intravitreal steroids such as Ozurdex may have a role. It must be stated however that local therapy must never be used instead of systemic therapy as VKH is a systemic disease and requires systemic treatment, but rather as an adjunct. In the acute stage, intravitreal therapy is risky and generally not advisable if there is still widespread subretinal fluid due to the risk of accidentally injecting the implant under the retina. However later in the course of the disease, when the fluid has disappeared, Ozurdex might play a role in decreasing the overall systemic steroid burden later in the course of disease and in controlling local ocular recurrences.

There is evidence that if you hit the disease 'early and hard' then you are more likely to get the disease into remission, while undertreatment will do the patient no favours and may sentence them to chronic disease. Another key point is that during therapy clinical examination alone may not be enough to be sure that the disease is entirely controlled, as there may not be any physical signs to see. FFA will be helpful here and assessing for subclinical active choroidal disease will be critical, with repeat ICG and enhanced depth OCT imaging. This also applies to sympathetic ophthalmia as these two diseases are two sides of the same coin. Even if the disease goes into remission the possibility of a recurrence is such that patients should be warned of this possibility and advised to get in touch immediately if this should occur. Never forget that even if VKH, or sympathetic ophthalmia, has been totally quiescent for many years you should always cover any planned intraocular procedure such as a cataract extraction with generous oral steroid before surgery, commonly prednisolone 60 mg od 5 days before surgery tapered by 5 mg decrements per week until it is discontinued, in order to reduce the chances of recurrence.

PLAQUE OF SCARRING EXTENDING FROM THE DISC ALONG THE VESSELS IN A PINCER MOVEMENT AROUND THE FOVEA: SERPIGINOUS CHOROIDITIS

Keeping with the theme of conditions with distinctive features we come to serpiginous choroiditis. Serpiginous means serpent-like or snake-like and this is in fact the perfect description for this. As with all bilateral conditions it can be highly asymmetric with one eye becoming involved years before the second. Classically there is a snake-like area of choroidal atrophy that starts at the optic disc and curls its way towards the fovea along the arcades in a highly variable pincer movement both superiorly and inferiorly (Figure 5.19). The affected area is a grey patch with a variably demarcated border and pigment disruption within it. It is a slow-burning constant fire so there is mild vitritis, if any, and never any anterior uveitis. Due to the very mild inflammation the patient can be asymptomatic until the pincer movement is complete and the fovea is involved, a process that can take months or years, or the condition can be picked up incidentally during routine examination. The borders of the affected area expand slowly and can sometimes skip small steps before the areas merge later on. It can take months or years until the fovea is destroyed. As with all conditions where there are atrophic scars, and this is a big atrophic scar, choroidal neovascularisation can form and become a problem of its own.

While 80% of all cases of serpiginous resemble Figure 5.19 there are other phenotypes to be aware of. **Macular serpiginous choroiditis** accounts for 10% of cases and is the most devastating version as the area of destruction can skip to the macula without waiting for the slow creep from the disc to take place (Figure 5.20). In a variant some call **ampiginous chorioretinitis** the condition resembles APMPPE with placoid lesions spread all over the fundus, but unlike APMPPE it does not settle spontaneously but goes on to behave in a serpiginous manner. Other variants have been described, but these are purely descriptive and do not really help our understanding.

When we see a patient with a serpiginous pattern of choroidal inflammation around either the optic disc or macula it is worth briefly examining the differential diagnosis. With the exception of tuberculous choroiditis, most other conditions are easy to distinguish. Sarcoidosis can present with choroidal involvement but there will usually be other features such as retinal vasculitis, retinitis or systemic features that give the game away. Likewise, a large toxoplasmosis scar can sometimes look 'serpiginous' but there will be other clues – if active, a very focal patch of chorioretinitis, overlying vitritis, surrounding vasculitis and often a hypertensive anterior uveitis. SLE with renovascular involvement and severe hypertension can cause choroidal

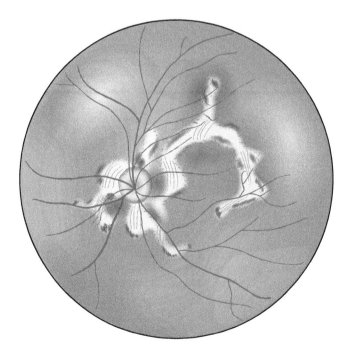

Figure 5.19 Serpiginous choroiditis.

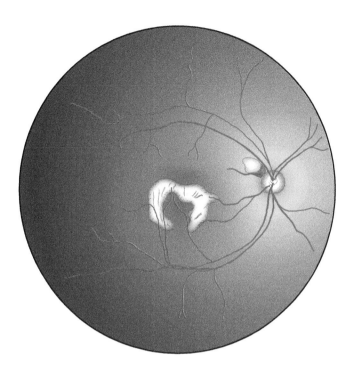

Figure 5.20 Macular serpiginous choroiditis.

infarcts that can look serpiginous, but the systemic features will give a clue. Syphilis can cause choroiditis in a form called **acute posterior placoid choroiditis** and therefore all patients with serpiginous choroiditis should be tested for this condition. Finally a very rare infection called tularaemia, a gram-negative coccobacillus, can cause a serpiginous choroiditis. Hunters who skin rabbits can be exposed to this infection, 'rabbit fever', which causes generalised sepsis with choroidal lesions. Interestingly an epidemic of tularaemia might have been the first recorded use of biological warfare, when it was deliberately introduced into western Anatolia during the Neshite-Arzawan conflict in the fourteenth-century BC, an epidemic termed the Hittite Plague.

While this is undoubtedly very interesting in reality the biggest challenge for the clinician will be distinguishing idiopathic choroiditis from tuberculous choroiditis. Clinically this appears indistinguishable from the idiopathic non-infectious form so a low threshold for suspecting this disease must be employed, particularly in endemic areas. Tuberculous choroiditis will therefore be a common cause of serpiginous choroiditis in Southeast Asia, the Indian subcontinent and in the West, usually in cities with large immigrant communities from these areas such as Hounslow in the west or Tower Hamlets in the east of London. You should have a low threshold for suspecting TB if you work in these areas and take a careful history, so always ask about TB exposure, a noteworthy cough in the past, fever or weight loss. All patients should have a chest X-ray but this is rarely helpful as more than 90% of them will be normal. Extensive searches for signs of chest disease are often futile as the ocular disease is usually an extrapulmonary manifestation and besides ophthalmologists should not be using the stethoscope in anger as we would be hard pressed to hear a nuclear explosion through standard issue National Health Service (NHS) devices, let alone the subtle signs of tuberculous infection.

QuantiFERON-TB Gold testing should be performed and although this has largely superseded the Mantoux test this can be useful if the QuantiFERON-TB Gold is negative but the disease is very strongly suspected and a medicolegal evidence base is needed to start the patient on potentially toxic anti-tuberculous therapy. The QuantiFERON-TB Gold alone cannot be totally relied upon as its sensitivity and specificity for predicting the response to TB therapy in the very particular case of TB choroiditis is low. We have seen patients with serpiginous uveitis and negative QuantiFERON-TB Gold tests respond well to anti-tuberculous therapy. If tuberculous choroiditis is suspected then the patient requires a course of full anti-TB therapy for 9–12 months, usually with systemic steroid cover to control the inflammation. For more on TB uveitis see the relevant section.

Once tuberculosis has been suspected and excluded, including syphilis if relevant, non-infectious, or idiopathic, serpiginous choroiditis can now be diagnosed and treated. This disease usually occurs between the ages of 30 and 50 years, with males and females equally affected. As already noted, anterior uveitis is almost never present, but a mild vitritis is common. The serpiginous features are identical to those previously described. If a patient with serpiginous choroiditis presents with acute deterioration the two possible causes include a choroidal neovascular (CNV) membrane and active inflammatory disease, encroaching the macula. FFA is traditionally used in demonstrating CNV, although OCT angiography is a non-invasive alternative which when the technology has developed may be useful in the future. Should a membrane be the cause FFA will demonstrate early well-defined hyperfluorescence in the area of the membrane but should active inflammation be the cause a far less well-defined fluffy hyperfluorescent border at the active edge is present. This distinction is important as the treatment for CNV in this context is an anti-VEGF injection, usually Avastin (bevacizumab) followed by a review 4 weeks later to see if another is warranted. The nature of the condition is such that CNV can form anywhere and if extramacular, photodynamic therapy (PDT) could be employed, though in practice it is intravitreal bevacizumab injections or nothing that is used.

A useful means of assessing whether the border of the serpiginous lesion is active is auto-fluorescence, which is a non-invasive means of assessing lesion activity. If active, then there is a bright border of increased autofluorescence at the edge of the serpiginous lesion, and this fades to hypo-autofluorescence when the lesion becomes inactive. Serial autofluorescence images will help you assess progression over time. OCT scanning is also very useful as in old inactive disease scarring is represented by discrete areas of well-defined reflectance and atrophy by thinned retina. Active disease on the other hand has a characteristic 'fluffy' border that is anything but well defined and the retina in the area of activity may be thickened and contain fluid.

The treatment of active inflammation is immunosuppression, usually in the form of oral prednisolone 60 mg for a week, 40 mg for a week, 30 mg for a week, 20 mg for a week, 15 mg for a week and 10 mg for a week with further treatment being dependent on the response. Long-term immunosuppression and the treatment of serpiginous choroiditis is controversial. Due to the chronic, relentless nature of the disease and stop-start small steps in scar progression with relatively minimal inflammation it is thought that aggressive immunosuppression with multiple steroid-sparing agents with or without biologics (Chapter 9) can result in a slowdown in disease progression but at a heavy price. Even with treatment, some progression is usual, to the extent that 25% of eyes end up with visual acuity of less than 6/60.

With the prognosis being so guarded it might be questioned what use there is in even trying to immunosuppress the patient in the long term. When the Luftwaffe was pounding London in the early days of the Blitz the ineffective anti-aircraft gun defence system was hopeless at hitting any of the high bombers but Prime Minister Winston Churchill ordered intensification of the firing rather than perhaps the more logical cessation, noting that the 'morale effect of the intensification of the AA barrage on the public has been very striking despite the lack of effect'. If a patient is inevitably going to eventually lose vision due to a condition such as serpiginous choroiditis they might feel much better having fought and tried something to save it, even if that effort was in vain, than do nothing and simply let it happen.

Finally, some authors have tried intravitreal steroid implants such as Ozurdex with modest success, primarily to reduce the burden of the systemic medications by enabling some systemic steroid lowering effect.

Tip: **Always test for TB in all cases of serpiginous choroiditis.**

EXTENSIVE SCARRING THROUGHOUT THE FUNDUS: PROGRESSIVE SUBRETINAL FIBROSIS AND UVEITIS SYNDROME

There is a severe variant of posterior uveitis believed to be in the same family as MCP. This rare condition is characterised by enlarging areas of sub-retinal fibrosis covering the fundus (Figure 5.21). It may be in patches, simulating very severe APMPPE scarring, or it may be in great plaques dominating the fundus. It is bilateral, though may be asymmetrical. It is notorious for failing to respond to steroids, conventional immunosuppressives and anti-TNF agents, and the prognosis historically has been very poor. Histological studies have shown that the inflammatory infiltrate is predominantly B cells and for this reason Rituximab (see Chapter 9) has been tried with better success.

A NEURORETINITIS: MACULAR STAR FORMATION WITH OPTIC DISC SWELLING

This is less a diagnosis and more a description of a specific clinical appearance of optic nerve head and peri-papillary swelling. A neurosensory detachment occurs with fluid and lipid

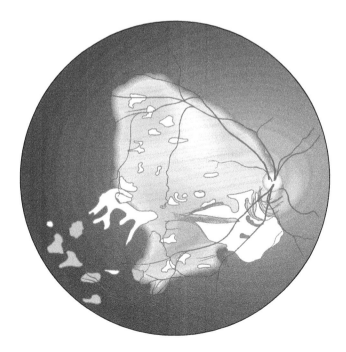

Figure 5.21 Progressive subretinal fibrosis and uveitis syndrome.

leaking intraretinally into Henle's layer giving the characteristic appearance of the macula star, which can be complete or incomplete. If severe, the lipid and exudate can track peripherally, far from the macula. The macula star can be present on presentation or can develop weeks later. This is the term 'neuro-retinitis' and because it represents an end pathology, there is a very long list of causes, which can be divided into inflammatory and non-inflammatory. Non-inflammatory causes include hypertension, raised intracranial pressure and diabetes, all of which must be thought of and looked for. Causes relevant to uveitis include infective causes such as cat scratch disease, syphilis, TB, Lyme disease, leptospirosis, toxoplasmosis and toxocariasis. Non-infective inflammatory causes include sarcoidosis, and a condition labelled recurrent idiopathic neuroretinitis.

The most celebrated cause of neuro-retinitis is cat scratch disease. This is caused by a bacterium called *Bartonella henselae*. As its name suggests the bacteria's main natural reservoir is the cat and the disease is spread from cat to cat and from cat to human by fleas, lice and other insects. It was once thought that a physical scratch was needed to transfer the bacteria but this is not true and there are plenty of cases reported in which no scratch has ever taken place, although the involvement of cats in some way is essential. It might be hypothesised that those cats most heavily infested with fleas might be more feral and more likely to lash out and scratch an approaching human. It can also be argued that cats are inherently selfish animals and almost all cat owners would get scratched at some point regardless of how feral the cat is.

There are many ways *Bartonella* can affect humans. Parinaud oculoglandular syndrome is one in which a unilateral conjunctivitis and lymphadenopathy can occur after infection. More rarely, a neuroretinitis can also occur and the classic textbook presentation of this is with a swollen disc and a macular star formed by exudates. The degree of uveitis, posterior or anterior, can vary considerably and although unilateral involvement is what is most commonly described there are reports of bilateral disease. The swollen disc appears first followed up to a month later by radial macular exudates resembling, and thus called, a macular star (see Figure 5.15). While the two previously mentioned conditions are potentially lethal cat scratch disease is typically similar to the annual cold or flu, though lymph nodes can become very tender and complications such as endocarditis and hepatitis can occur. Being infectious rather than inflammatory if no treatment were undertaken the condition can resolve though it may take months and leave permanent scars which would have been avoided had antibiotics been given.

This clinical picture is typical of cat scratch though rarely Lyme disease, caused by the spirochete *Borrelia burgdorferi* spread by deer ticks, can also present this way. Malignant hypertension and diabetic retinopathy are both known for exudates and swollen discs though these would almost always be bilateral, and syphilis can masquerade as anything. Tests in this scenario would include **Bartonella and Borrelia serology, syphilis serology, blood pressure** and **serum glucose**. Serology here is neither sensitive nor very specific so must be reserved for cases where this diagnosis is truly considered. In fact the UK government laboratory responsible for carrying out serology has recently closed and serum samples must be processed privately or sent to France. Only order this test if absolutely necessary as quite apart from the cost, great confusion can result. Much ado is made about the cross-reactivity of the serum *Bartonella* test with other similar organisms such as the one responsible for trench fever but seeing as the First World War ended a hundred years ago this is purely of academic interest.

While it is true that mild cat scratch disease need not be treated at all, if posterior uveitis with vasculitis is present treatment is obviously needed. Doxycycline 100 mg po bd for 2 weeks should be given in adults but due to the risk of tooth staining and growth retardation in children erythromycin 500 mg twice a day should be used here, which is also an alternative option in adults. Should an anterior uveitis be present, treatment is with topical steroids as described in Chapter 3. Should the posterior uveitis be severe it seems logical to consider a short course of oral steroids as well although it is prudent to consider whether the patient is immunosuppressed if the posterior uveitis is very bad and if there is a lot of vitritis.

Should the serum Borreliosis test return positive and **Lyme disease** be suspected it is prudent to ask one or two questions:

Question 1: Have you been to any woods, hunted deer or been hiking recently?
Question 2: Have you had any skin rashes or been bitten by anything?

If the answer to these two questions is no then Lyme disease is unlikely. If one or both answers are yes then Lyme disease needs to be suspected and a referral to the physicians undertaken for treatment with intravenous ceftriaxone for 3 weeks. The physicians should lead this as there are other organs, such as the heart especially, that could be involved and could result in a life-threatening emergency.

In terms of other non-infectious inflammatory causes of neuroretinitis, only a few warrant mention: sarcoidosis, idiopathic retinal vasculitis and neuroretinitis (IRVAN) syndrome and idiopathic neuroretinitis (INR). In sarcoidosis there are usually other features of ocular sarcoid or other systemic manifestations. IRVAN is described above.

Idiopathic neuroretinitis (INR) is worth knowing about as although it is a diagnosis of exclusion, in our practice it is the most common non-infectious cause of neuroretinitis. INR usually occurs in young adults with more than half reporting a preceding flu-like illness. Most cases are unilateral and the INR is typically painless; significant pain, or bilateral disease should prompt a search for an alternative diagnosis such as posterior scleritis. The presenting vision is typically in the region of 6/18–6/60, but can be normal, or severely impaired. It is important to understand that the visual loss is primarily due to macular involvement rather than true optic nerve dysfunction. In this sense it differs from demyelinating disease and it is important to explain to the patient that in confirmed INR there is no increased risk of multiple sclerosis. Patients are often treated in the acute stage with a tapering course of oral steroids. Some patients develop recurrent attacks, with the interval between attacks varying from a month to many years, but with a mean of 3 years. Patients with frequent attacks can be treated with long-term immunosuppressive therapy, which has been shown to reduce the frequency of recurrent attacks.

IS THERE A HIDDEN CAUSE OF POSTERIOR UVEITIS PRESENT?

We turn now to the last question we ask in categorising posterior uveitis. To get to this point we have ascertained that the patient has various symptoms of posterior uveitis but on first examination there is no sight-threatening pathology, no dots or spots, no vasculitis and no other distinguishing feature. In fact the eye looks normal. It is at this point that some people panic and diagnose a posterior vitreous detachment or some other pathology just to mollify the patient and get on with the clinic. Some will be honest and say they can see nothing wrong. There are specific diagnoses that should be considered in just this scenario however, and we go through them one by one.

ACUTE IDIOPATHIC BLIND SPOT ENLARGEMENT SYNDROME

AIBSE is an intriguing condition thought to be related to MEWDS (see above) in some as yet unspecified way, and could be looked at as MEWDS without the dots, which are hard to see anyway. Essentially, young myopic women present with unilateral photopsia and a scotoma, usually described as being in the temporal field, with dilated fundal examination often being normal, at least in the early stages. A RAPD might have been spotted had this been undertaken before dilation, though due to the symptoms the patient is usually dilated by the time this diagnosis is first considered. A Humphrey 24-2 field test will reveal a unilaterally enlarged blind spot. In fact, it is the visual field result that lets you diagnose this condition, and it is an essential diagnostic test. Fundus autofluorescence is also very helpful, as this non-invasive test will show a distinct halo of increased autofluorescence (hyper-autofluorescence) around the optic disc, and there is corresponding loss of the ellipsoid layer in this area that can be identified with spectral domain OCT imaging.

There is a prodromal flu-like illness in a significant number of people beforehand and there is no effective treatment. As with MEWDS the condition can rarely be bilateral and it might be sensible to think of AIBSE, MEWDS and contentiously even acute zonal occult outer retinopathy (AZOOR) (see below) as being on a spectrum of severity. This corner of uveitis is much like chemistry before Dmitri Mendeleev organised his periodic table. There are competing theories with some uveitis specialists keen to split off and organise groups of signs and symptoms into distinct entities, while others lump all the similar things together into a mystic stew, which is fascinating as it implies unity but is not really helpful to the ophthalmologist faced with a patient. In practice it is best to reassure the patient with AIBSE that the condition is unlikely to worsen, that there is no treatment needed, and to follow up with a repeat visual field test, and imaging, in around 4 months.

ACUTE ZONAL OCCULT OUTER RETINOPATHY

If MEWDS and AIBSE had a big brother, this would be it. It is convenient to think of it as AIBSE plus another patch of affected retina which can be any size and located away from the disc. It is much more common in Caucasian women, usually in their 30s or 40s, and presents with photopsia and a scotoma, with the photopsia being universal in AZOOR as opposed to occurring in the majority of AIBSE patients. In fact the photopsia is striking in that it is invariably described as an intrusive glittering or shimmering that is made worse by bright light. Again there is commonly a prodromal illness. Unilateral involvement is the classic presentation but ultimately 75% eventually end up with bilateral disease. A Humphrey 24-2 field test is valuable as it will always show a visual field defect, though the defect can be variable and does not always fit a pattern. An enlarged blind spot may be seen along with a visual field defect approximating to the involved area of retina. If unilateral an RAPD of varying severity will be present, and though this is classically less pronounced than that present in AIBSE this is far from being a hard and fast rule.

When first presenting, as the 'occult' in the name suggests, there is not much to be seen. The anterior chamber (AC) is quiet and on cursory inspection the vitreous appears quiet. Careful inspection might show the occasional vitreous cell, usually in the posterior vitreous, and in the region of the affected retina. Very occasionally there is a thin white demarcation line between the area of affected retina and the rest, which if photographs are taken on subsequent days can be seen to move slowly before disappearing altogether. If an OCT scan is taken through this border the contrast between the healthy and the neighbouring atrophic outer retina is striking. This line is only seen in a minority, however. A fundus autofluorescence picture will easily demonstrate the affected area as an area of hypo-autofluorescence, which the human eye cannot see, bringing what is occult out into the open. After a few months to years the funduscopic view will also change as the affected area begins to resemble a sectoral retinitis pigmentosa, with bone spicule pigmentation and attenuated vessels. Investigation wise syphilis serology is advised, as well as a field test and fundus autofluorescence picture, which if available is best performed as a wide-field picture to capture peripheral involvement. In the late stages the FFA and ICG begin to show signs of abnormality but by and large in the acute phase these are normal and not useful.

Tip: **If a patient presents with photopsia and an apparently normal retinal exam, AZOOR can be easily investigated with a Humphrey visual field and wide-field autofluorescence.**

Electrodiagnostic testing reveals abnormalities including a reduced ERG, a delayed 30 Hz flicker, a sub-normal pattern electroretinogram (PERG) in the case of macular involvement and characteristically a sub-normal electro-oculogram (EOG). For many clinicians, an abnormal electrodiagnostic test is essential in making the diagnosis, particularly given the subtlety of the clinical signs.

The prognosis of AZOOR is rather variable and depends on whether the fovea has been involved as well as how much of the periphery has been affected, with some patients exhibiting spontaneous remission. There is no clear evidence of any treatment that has stabilised or improved visual function and all sorts of therapies have been tried, generally with poor results. Therapies that have been tried include steroids, with or without immunosuppression, most other immunomodulatory therapies, antifungals and antivirals. All have disappointing results. Given the absence of any convincing evidence of an effective treatment, it is reasonable to at least demonstrate progression with objective evidence such as visual fields or electrodiagnostic tests before contemplating any therapy. A course of steroids, with or without immunosuppression, could be tried though it would be reasonable to choose the agent with the fewest potential side effects. *Primum non nocere* – 'first do no harm'.

ACUTE MACULAR NEURORETINOPATHY

If AZOOR is AIBSE's big brother then AMN might be considered a smaller cousin. The typical case involves a young woman with unilateral small para-central scotoma of sudden onset. Prof. Bird of Moorfields Eye Hospital in London states that the giveaway sign is that the patient insists on drawing the scotoma for the ophthalmologist and should the doctor remove all pen and paper the patient will then carve the scotoma she sees onto the tabletop in front of her. While this is obviously not true in the strict sense there does seem to be anecdotal agreement among medical retina specialists about AMN patients carrying little bits of paper with a perfectly drawn scotoma to their appointments. The visual acuity and examination of the fundus is almost always entirely normal and traditionally the patient would have been told all is well and discharged, or given some other diagnosis to get her to leave the room. Any patient presenting with a sudden scotoma and an accompanying piece of paper with a scotoma drawn on it should be thought to have AMN until proven otherwise.

Not all eye departments have spectral domain optical coherence tomography, such a Spectralis OCT machine, but if it is possible to perform one an abnormality will be demonstrated at the inner segment/outer segment junction corresponding to the scotoma. Infrared autofluorescence can also map the affected retina. This condition is almost certainly underdiagnosed but an argument could be made that it matters not if this is the case as there is no treatment that can be given and the scotoma almost never resolves, never threatens vision and almost always changes little if at all over extended periods of time. Perhaps one day more information will be available on what causes this condition and how to treat it but until then the patient should be reassured and discharged.

CANCER-ASSOCIATED RETINOPATHY

Although this paraneoplastic syndrome is extremely rare, patients present with similar symptoms, hence the mention here. Patients complain of significant photopsia, photophobia and acute painless loss of vision. Symptoms are bilateral but can be asymmetric and suggestive of both cone involvement (visual acuity loss, colour disturbance and central scotoma) and rod involvement (peripheral field loss and impaired dark adaptation). In keeping with the theme of these diseases in the initial stages the examination will be normal. In late disease a retinal appearance similar to AZOOR can develop. It is thought to be due to a tumour-related immune response in which antibodies are created which cross-react with retinal proteins. Continuing the similarity with AZOOR, abnormal visual fields, fundus autofluorescence and outer segment loss on OCT will be present. Electrodiagnostic testing is key for the diagnosis and will always demonstrate abnormalities, usually of both rod and cone dysfunction. Cancer-associated retinopathy (CAR) is one of the rare causes of an 'electronegative' ERG but this phenomenon is far more common with melanoma-associated retinopathy (MAR – see below).

In more than 90% of cases the patient will present with CAR after a known diagnosis of malignancy, often at metastatic stage. If however the patient does not have any history of cancer the ophthalmologist must ask about any weight loss, bowel, breast or gynaecological symptoms. Should the patient admit to any problem with any system an urgent referral must be made to that specialty. Always ask about skin cancers, and in particular melanoma (see below) in this situation. It is not recommended that we perform our own examination of body systems we are unfamiliar with in the open environment of the eye clinic. At best we would not find any useful information and at worst we might end up with a General Medical Council referral. If there is absolutely nothing pointing towards a cancer of any system then a referral to oncologists is warranted, and they can perform a malignancy screen looking for an overt or occult malignancy. The prognosis is poor, usually because there is irreversible photoreceptor loss by the time the diagnosis is confirmed. Treatments with steroid, either alone or combined with immunosuppression, have been tried with disappointing results. For obvious reasons it is best to liaise with the physicians and the oncologists before suppressing the immune system of a cancer patient. Occasional success has been reported with plasmapheresis, with visual improvement reported if the treatment is started early in the course of the disease.

MELANOMA-ASSOCIATED RETINOPATHY

This is a subset of CAR in which the patient has had a melanoma of the skin removed in the past. Compared to CAR, symptoms are similar but often milder, and at presentation the acuity is better. The fundus examination is equally normal looking, but the autofluorescence and OCT changes are the same as CAR. Happily from a diagnostic standpoint the melanoma is almost always pre-existing, although if the patient has no history of this it might be worth asking if they have noticed any recent changes to any skin lesions. If the patient has not then as mentioned above it is inappropriate for us to ask the patient to strip and go hunting ourselves for suspicious lesions. Should the patient admit to a lesion then urgent referral to a dermatologist is advised.

Investigation is exactly as with CAR, and again the ERG is a very useful test to perform. Characteristically the ERG is electronegative here, and MAR is one of celebrated causes of an 'electronegative' ERG, but it is not the only cause (see Table 5.16). The treatment strategy is similar to that for CAR.

Table 5.16 Causes of an electronegative electroretinogram

Melanoma-associated retinopathy (MAR) and rarely cancer-associated retinopathy (CAR)
X-linked juvenile retinoschisis
Congenital stationary night blindness
Central retinal artery obstruction
Ischaemic central retinal vein occlusion
Birdshot, and other non-specific inflammatory retinopathies
Batten disease
Myotonic dystrophy
Drug toxicity – quinine and vigabatrin

THE END OF THE ALGORITHM

We have now reached the end of the five-question algorithm. Posterior uveitis in particular is notorious for being complicated and nebulous and while in truth much of it still is we hope that this guide has gone some way towards making order out of chaos. Posterior uveitis is like the Wild West; gradually over time inroads will be made, new towns set up, roads and railways laid down and civilisation will come as counties and then states are cleaved away from the wilderness to make organised, accountable entities. For now territories are still being carved out or re-classified: one important senator proposes a state incorporating much of the West and another proposes a smaller state encompassing the settled land alone. Up and coming lawmen and sheriffs propose to split counties into two due to perceived differences and a large enough population to support two separate councils. If a logical approach is taken, however, then the ophthalmologists can get themselves to California in one piece.

All the conditions covered in this chapter are diagnosable based on this algorithm but what of a uveitis so severe that no details are visible? What if the inflammation obscures the retinal view to such an extent that no questions can be answered? This condition is called panuveitis and this will be dealt with next.

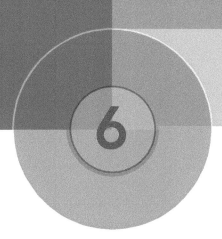

Panuveitis

6

We come now to inflammation so severe that the algorithm in Chapter 5 cannot be used. The fundus is not visible enough to enable details such as spots, dots, vasculitis or indeed any features whatsoever to guide the ophthalmologist. At this point it is easy to panic and lose track of basic principles but in a way panuveitis is even simpler to investigate and manage than a posterior uveitis as the very lack of information simplifies things immeasurably. As we saw in Chapter 5 a great number of posterior uveities can cause a panuveitis, but the majority of those usually allow a decent enough view of the fundus so that the algorithm can be put into effect. There are a relatively small number of pathologies that cloud the vitreous so much as to make any meaningful interpretation of the state of the retina impossible. Table 6.1 lists these causes.

The great tomes of inflammatory eye disease list a further 10 or so inflammatory causes rather than lump everything into the last on Table 6.1, but in practice this is unnecessary as the treatment initially is the same and as the condition improves a greater view of the fundus can help guide more specific treatment. There are a few questions that can guide us as to which of the five points in Table 6.1 is the likely culprit, too:

Question 1: Have you had any recent eye surgery, had any injury to the eye or had any severe infection elsewhere like a joint or in the stomach?

If the answer is yes then infectious endophthalmitis will be high on the list.

Question 2: Have you ever had an infection called 'toxoplasmosis' in the eye that flares up from time to time?

A raised intraocular pressure will also point in this direction.

Question 3: Do you have any medical condition that causes inflammation of joints, skin or other organs?

Question 4: Don't worry, we ask these questions to everyone with an inflamed eye like this. How many sexual partners have you had in the past 6 months? Were they men, women or both? Are you having protected or unprotected sex?

This last question, clearly designed to see if syphilis may be the causative agent, is seldom answered truthfully at the first asking but is always worth trying. You will be in one of two positions at this point – with a clue as to what the cause is or without. The obvious one to deal with first is infectious endophthalmitis.

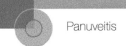
Table 6.1 Most common causes of panuveitis with absolutely no fundal view

Pathology
Acute retinal necrosis
Toxoplasmosis
Syphilis
Infectious endophthalmitis
An inflammatory cause

INFECTIOUS ENDOPHTHALMITIS

As the name suggests this is an infection inside the eyeball causing inflammation. A recent history of eye surgery of any variety will point in this direction. So as not to be overwhelmed by all this a few key considerations can be borne in mind in the correct order which will guide us in the right direction.

Is this an endophthalmitis? If so, what is the likely causative pathogen?

Key consideration 1: Over what time period has the disease progressed?

Any endophthalmitis that rapidly progresses over the course of hours to a day or so should be considered bacterial until proven otherwise. Furthermore, such devastating clinical worsening over hours is a characteristic of ß-haemolytic streptococci, and to a lesser extent *Pseudomonas*. In contrast, fungal, viral and other 'low-grade' bacterial infections such as Propionibacterium acnes infections progress much more slowly. Typically highly pathogenic bacterial infections will be associated with lid swelling, massive chemosis, corneal oedema and have severe signs of intraocular inflammation such as a hypopyon and dense vitritis. It is not unusual for such patients to present with severe elevation of intraocular pressure. The fundal view is usually absent, but if present white haemorrhagic retinal infiltrates, serous detachments and disc swelling may be seen. If no fundal view is possible, which is usually the case, B-scan ultrasound will show dense vitreous debris, possibly with serous retinal detachment and thickening of the posterior coats. A grossly enlarged ciliary body is a distinctive B-scan finding that has been described in streptococcal endophthalmitis in particular.

Key consideration 2: Is this exogenous or endogenous?

This is a critical distinction. **Exogenous** endophthalmitis is a consequence of the spread of micro-organisms as a direct result of inoculation through the external coat of the eye. In all cases there will be a clue or pre-disposing factor. This complication can occur after trauma, any form of intraocular surgery, an intravitreal injection, in association with tube implants or buckle explants, or as sequelae of a severe keratitis. On rare occasions, we have seen devastating exogenous group B streptococcal endophthalmitis present without a predisposing factor other than severe blepharitis.

    Endogenous endophthalmitis in reality means haematogenous spread from any infected source elsewhere in the body. This is one of those times where ophthalmologists need to remember that the eye is connected to other organs. A patient with a mysterious eye inflammation who hobbled in to clinic with great difficulty on account of his suddenly painful hip that had been causing trouble for the preceding week attended more than twice before the two things were connected. Common sense and taking a thorough history should alert the ophthalmologist to any recent history of sepsis. There are a few risk factors that must be remembered such as patient who has had recent hospital admission, diabetes, a previous history of recent intravenous cannulation, IV drug abusers and women in the early post-partum period. Other risk factors are those patients with heart valve disease, particularly those with prosthetic valves, or indeed any other prosthesis.

Post-operative endophthalmitis tends to present a few days to a week after the eye surgery has taken place. The most common organism is skin flora; *Staphylococcus epidermidis* and *Staphylococcus aureus*, though *Streptococcus* can also make a rarer appearance. There is worsening pain and very poor vision with examination revealing a panuveitis. The anterior component is usually severe with a hypopyon while the posterior segment may have such a dense vitritis that visualisation of the fundus is impossible.

Irrespective of whether the endophthalmitis is endogenous or exogenous this condition needs to be **treated as an emergency**. All patients need an urgent vitreous tap and injection of antibiotics, called a 'tap and inject'. Prior to this a B-scan ultrasound is traditionally carried out at this point to see if the retina is detached. While a B-scan can be helpful to assess the posterior segment, if endophthalmitis is suspected do not delay a 'tap and inject' while you wait for this investigation if not immediately available. Retinal detachment is rare in endopthalmitis pre-tap. You should, however, arrange for a B-scan of all patients within 24–48 hours post-tap, if not performed beforehand.

The 'tap and inject' can be performed in a clean room, for example in a minor ops room, or at the end of a theatre or intravitreal list. You should not delay awaiting a theatre slot if not immediately available. The antibiotics injected consist of ceftazidime 2 mg in 0.1 mL to cover the gram-negative organisms and vancomycin 1 mg in 0.1 mL to cover the gram-positives, though amikacin 0.4 mg in 0.1 mL is sometimes used as an alternative to ceftazidime. The antibiotics can be prepared in 1 mL syringes with fine needles (27–30 G). If you prepare the injections yourself remember to take double the volume (i.e. 0.2 mL) when drawing up, and then push the plunger down to the 0.1 mark in order to allow for the dead-space. It takes a while to get these concentrations just right and the pharmacy must be contacted in plenty of time so that they are ready for use at the time of the procedure. In some places there is an 'out of hours' box consisting of the materials necessary to produce the appropriate concentration and volume of drugs needed and it feels a bit like an episode of *Breaking Bad* following the instructions to get the right dose. It can take up to 20 minutes to do it right so leave plenty of time if this is being done out of hours. This is how a traditional 'tap and inject' is performed:

1. Perform the procedure in a clean room, or in theatre at the end of a list or out of hours.
2. Place oxybuprocaine drops in the patient's eye, followed by 5% iodine, as per preparation for an intravitreal injection.
3. Apply 10% iodine skin preparation, followed by a sterile drape and speculum.
4. Apply another drop of oxybuprocaine. For additional anaesthesia, you can apply a cotton bud soaked in Tetracaine against the conjunctiva for a minute at the planned site of tap (inferotemporally is easiest).
5. Advance a 1 mL syringe and orange needle (25 gauge) into the vitreous 4 mm posterior to the limbus (phakic eye) or 3.5 mm (pseudophakic or aphakic eye) and withdraw at least 0.3 mL of fluid. It is best to get a generous sample.
6. Usually in cases of endophthalmitis the vitreous is liquefied, and may even be purulent, so it is usually easy to get a sample. If this is not possible, a 'dry tap', try gently advancing the needle, turning the bevel or angling the needle slightly posteriorly. Failing this withdrawing and repeating the procedure with a blue needle (23 gauge) can be considered. If it is still not possible do not persist.

7. Gently detach the syringe from the needle, leaving the needle in place in the eye, and pass to an assistant so that a sterile cap can be placed. If this is fiddly or gives you grey hairs gently remove the needle and syringe together and pass to an assistant so that a sterile cap can be placed.

8. You now need to inject the two intravitreal antibiotics. If the needle is still in place you can gently attach each syringe in turn to inject 0.1 mL of the two antibiotics. If the needle is removed you will notice that the eye is now very soft post-tap so counterpressure is needed with a cotton bud on the globe 90–180° away from the site to give the eye a little pressure. Short intravitreal needles will help here. Gently inject 0.1 mL of the two antibiotics in the same area as the tap. They cannot be placed in the same syringe as a precipitation reaction can occur.

9. Remove the speculum and drape and clean the eye.

10. Prepare the sample for transport to the laboratory. Each hospital has a different procedure and it is paramount to check beforehand how the microbiology team want the sample. As this is a post-operative endophthalmitis the entire sample can be sent for culture and sensitivity.

Consider also doing an anterior chamber (AC) tap as 20% of patients have a culture-positive aqueous when the vitreous sample is negative though if performed it must be done after the main vitreous sample as the eye will be left in a very soft state, making the vitreous sampling very hazardous. This can be performed using a 27-gauge (grey) intravitreal needle and the procedure is discussed in Chapter 2. If in doubt omit the AC tap. Finally, if there is a severe fibrinous reaction in the AC consider injecting recombinant tissue plasminogen activator (rTPA) 25 micrograms in 0.05 mL, diluted with balanced salt solution (BSS), into the AC after the AC tap. This is very effective in breaking down the fibrin and will facilitate the fundal view, though it is difficult to obtain in some units.

Treatment wise the patient is started **on topical Maxidex (dexamethasone 0.1%) steroid drops** to be given at **hourly** intervals throughout the day and a cycloplegic in the form of **cyclopentolate 1% one drop twice a day**. Topical antibiotics really have no role in the treatment of typical endophthalmitis, though exceptions include trabeculectomy-related 'blebitis' with pus in a thin-walled bleb or a corneal suture related abscess that has progressed to endophthalmitis. Topical antibiotics are occasionally started four times a day (qds) as some sort of post-tap infection prophylaxis but there is no real need. Traditionally oral antibiotics are also started but this was more to benefit the doctor that everything was being done rather than conferring any actual useful benefit to the patient. Ciprofloxacin 750 mg twice daily (bd) is the most common oral antibiotic. An alternative is oral Moxifloxacin 400 mg od, but this must not be used in children, or anyone with a history of liver disease. Likewise most specialists start oral prednisolone at this point on the basis that it calms the inflammation faster although again in practice while this may be so there is no real effect on the end visual acuity. A starting dose of prednisolone 60 mg once daily (od) can be commenced within 24 hours post-tap, as long as fungal endophthalmitis is not suspected.

The patient should be reviewed in 2 days and if improving the current treatment continued. If worsening a repeat of the intravitreal injection of antibiotic should be considered, ideally combined with vitrectomy. To gauge 'worsening' we rely on signs such as worsening vision, for example from counting fingers to perception of light; worsening pain, or worsening anterior segment signs. This might manifest as increasing AC fibrin and increasing hypopyon. By this stage the Gram stain and potentially early microbiology results are back to guide treatment. A repeat second intravitreal antibiotic injection should only be given once a B-scan has excluded retinal detachment. At this stage, discuss the case with your local vitreoretinal specialists as an emergency vitrectomy can be beneficial, and the VR surgeons can perform an AC washout, a core vitrectomy and deliver a repeat intravitreal antibiotic after their procedure. In such severe cases, the vision will be very poor, and the end outcome is usually quite bad despite the best efforts of the ophthalmologist and the patient should be prepared for the worst from the beginning. On occasion, we have seen impressive and remarkable visual recovery following early vitrectomy, but this is rarely seen in patients who receive repeated intravitreal antibiotic injections alone.

Improvement is usually frustratingly slow and it takes weeks for the inflammation to settle. However the pain, which can be severe on presentation, should settle quickly following the 'tap and inject' and failure to do so would be unusual. Oral steroids do speed up this process though as must be emphasised again do not improve the end visual acuity; if used the dose is 60 mg for a week, 40 mg for a week, 30 mg for a week, 20 mg for a week and 10 mg for a week, before the steroids are discontinued. Oral lansoprazole 30 mg or omeprazole 20 mg should be concurrently given. It is customary to wait for stabilisation before steroids are started as the fear is that immunosuppression in the face of active infection would make the infection worse. There is no evidence for this however, in fact no evidence either way for anything, with some ophthalmologists starting steroids immediately at presentation and some even injecting steroid at the time of initial vitreous tap and inject. We would not advocate this however. The view of the fundus takes weeks to reappear and even then the debris obscures the view a great deal. It is not uncommon to refer the patient for a vitrectomy many weeks after the infection simply to clear this debris, commonly called a 'cold vitrectomy'.

If the infection has arrived in the eye via haematogenous spread from a source elsewhere the initial ophthalmic treatment is exactly the same as described above. Post-'tap and inject', an immediate referral needs to be made to the relevant medical team, and this must take priority, as in fact the eye is only a manifestation of potential systemic sepsis, which can potentially be life threatening. If the source of the infection is obvious then refer to the relevant specialty; for example orthopaedic surgeons in the case of an infected hip prosthesis, but if not refer to the general physicians who can then look for the source of sepsis. Systemic steroids could make a systemic infection worse if sepsis is present and they should be absolutely avoided until the physicians decree it is safe to use them, if they are to be used at all. The prognosis for recovery of good vision following endogenous endophthalmitis is not great.

Low-grade postoperative endophthalmitis, while not causing a fundus obscuring panuveitis is a post-operative infection which causes grumbling low-grade anterior uveitis. This is usually lumped into the 'post-operative uveitis' box in eye casualty and treated with topical steroids, which transiently improve things, with the situation deteriorating again on stopping the steroids. Several cycles of this should convince the ophthalmologist that all may not be as it seems. If this happens after a cataract operation the tell-tale sign is of white plaques on the lens and posterior capsule. A common mistake here is for the poor vision to be put down to 'posterior capsule opacification', and for an yttrium aluminium garnet (YAG) laser capsulotomy to be performed which then converts a grumbling chronic anterior uveitis into a true panuveitis as the organism now has free access to the posterior segment. Classically (and for exam purposes) Propionibacterium acnes is the cause of this, as any organism more virulent would cause an acute infectious endophthalmitis proper. Due to the biofilm on an artificial intraocular surface a 'tap and inject' almost never works and early referral to a vitreoretinal surgeon is prudent. The best procedure is an intraocular lens explant, vitrectomy and removal of the posterior capsule, if not already lasered, followed by injection of antibiotic and secondary implant of a sulcus lens at a later date when the infection has settled.

This should not be confused with 'UGH syndrome'. This stands for **uveitis glaucoma hyphaema syndrome** and is a form of low-grade chronic post-cataract operation uveitis which results from chafing of the lens on the iris. This can be due to inappropriate placement such as using a one-piece lens in the sulcus, or be due to tilting inside the capsule or other sequelae caused by anatomical variation or surgical technique. Retroillumination of the iris shows areas of atrophy where the actual chafing is taking place. As with chronic post-operative endophthalmitis the only solution is a lens explant.

FUNGAL ENDOPHTHALMITIS

This is the best moment to discuss fungal endophthalmitis. Patients with this condition are typically very unwell and junior ophthalmologists may be asked to see the patient on the ward or in intensive care as organisms have been found on blood culture. The typical patient has needed inpatient medical care for a month or more, has catheters, long lines or other medical paraphernalia attached to the body and is systemically unwell from any of a variety of reasons. As discussed above, infectious endophthalmitis from bacterial sources can arrive at the eye via haematogenous spread and the same is true for fungi. It is fairly unusual to develop fungal endophthalmitis following eye surgery. Armed with an indirect ophthalmoscope, some dilating drops and a 20 D lens the ophthalmologist enters the intensive care unit with trepidation, armed with the knowledge that the more critically unwell the patient the greater is the chance of discovering ocular signs of fungal infection.

Though highly immunosuppressed patients such as those suffering from acquired immune deficiency syndrome (AIDS) can develop a smorgasbord of weird and wonderful infections in the eye, the only two to truly know about in real life are *Candida* and *Aspergillus*. The presence of fungal endophthalmitis should therefore prompt an **HIV test** should another obvious cause of immunosuppression be lacking. *Candida* is a yeast and is ubiquitous among humanity with the great majority of us carrying it around as a commensal. As it reaches the eye through haematogenous spread the first appearance may be as a deep choroidal or subretinal mass. The organism is not aggressive and progress takes weeks rather than days and should treatment not be undertaken it will break through the retinal pigment epithelium (RPE) to form the typical white fluffy retinal lesions (Figure 6.1) that this condition is known for. If still left untreated the inward growth of *Candida* continues and the vitreous is entered, where it forms a 'string of pearls' that sits proud of the retina and seems to be joined together by a thin strand of fungal debris (Figure 6.2). Further progression causes the vitreous to fill with colonies and gliotic reaction to the presence of the invader can result in a tractional retinal detachment which can be impossible to repair. For this reason intensive care physicians will call ophthalmologists to examine all of their patients with positive *Candida* blood cultures. The key lies in capturing the infection early.

Should the infection be caught when the fungus is still in the retina or choroid, treatment with oral agents such as fluconazole 200 mg bd or voriconazole, also 200 mg bd for up to 6 weeks may do the trick, after initial loading of 400 mg bd for the first day, though consultation with local microbiologists and the intensive care physician is needed before starting anything. They will also plan the removal of any continuous sources of infection such as long lines or catheters but it may be helpful to mention this to them upon diagnosis of ocular candidiasis. Should the organism be suspected of being resistant, intravenous therapy with amphotericin B may be used, though as the dose is dependent upon weight and the other medications the patient is being administered, this should again be a suggestion to the team looking after the patient rather than something started by the ophthalmologists without consultation.

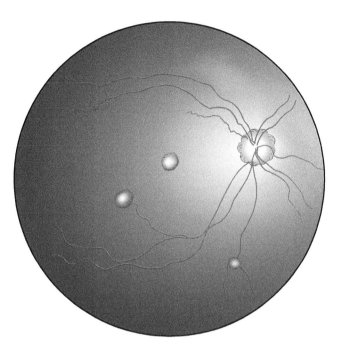

Figure 6.1 Ocular candidiasis before breakthrough into the vitreous.

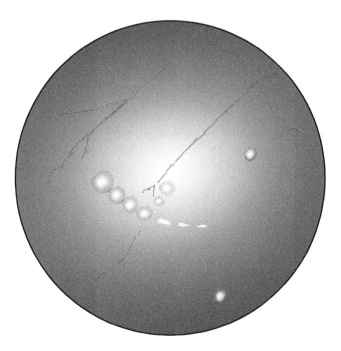

Figure 6.2 Ocular candidiasis after breakthrough into the vitreous.

If the fungus has reached the vitreous, systemic treatment alone will almost never suffice. In the first instance an intravitreal injection of 5 micrograms of amphotericin B in 0.1 mL or 25 micrograms voriconazole in 0.1 mL can be given though the nature of the typical patient is such that arranging for administration in an intensive care setting is challenging at best. Drawing up the exact concentration is essential, as too concentrated a dose can cause significant retinal damage. Liaising with pharmacy is vital for getting the dose exactly right. The truth is that the worse the vitreous involvement, the less likely injections are to work in which case the only option is to perform a vitrectomy. Patients can be too unwell for this, however, which presents a quandary. What commonly happens is that the ophthalmologists delay due to the systemic condition and anxiously watch the eye worsen while waiting for the intensive care physicians to approve surgery, while injecting the eye with toxic antifungals in the meantime in a bid to keep the forces of darkness at bay. These injections can be repeated if needed at weekly intervals but no more frequently. The progress of the disease is such that weekly review is more than sufficient as well.

It is possible, of course, that a patient who is not a hospital inpatient or with a known diagnosis of candidiasis presents with a fungal endophthalmitis but again they would need to be systemically unwell and there must always be a cause, such as intravenous drug abuse or AIDS, to explain it. Here a sample must be taken to confirm the diagnosis, and if this is considered we can use one stone to kill two birds by undertaking a vitrectomy to remove the fungus, as the waste fluid can be sent to the laboratory. A patient who walks into clinic would be more likely to endure a vitrectomy than a debilitated patient already admitted to hospital for a while.

While candidiasis is by far the most common cause of fungal endophthalmitis there are others of which **aspergillosis** is the most common. Aspergillus is not a normal commensal organism and as such is more aggressive and thus the patient does not need to be as debilitated to be affected by it, although people with AIDS and chronic lung diseases such as chronic obstructive pulmonary disease (COPD) are more likely to be affected than completely healthy people. The usual entry point to the human body is via the lungs and a chest x-ray can reveal a mass termed an 'aspergilloma' where the first colony grew after infection. Other organs may be affected before the eye, or afterwards, and as soon as this diagnosis is suspected referral must be made immediately to the physicians or infectious disease specialists to manage the systemic manifestations. Almost always however others have made this diagnosis before us and our role is to comfortably deal with the only organ we truly understand: the eye. The fundal view is similar to candidiasis though as the organism is more aggressive there is more inflammation and there is a tendency for one or two chorioretinal masses to dominate rather than having multiple discreet smaller lesions (Figure 6.3). As the growth is faster and the organism is more aggressive the lesions have areas of haemorrhage within them and a vitreous haemorrhage, even obscuring the fundal view, can occur.

The treatment is the same as with candidiasis above although all cases should be given intravitreal antifungal injections with a vitrectomy performed as soon as is practicable. Close liaison with the physicians is essential. There are many other fungi that can affect the eyes though knowledge of each one of these is more confusing than beneficial. The principles of investigation and treatment of unknown ocular fungi are the same where knowledge of the systemic condition, any growths from blood cultures and the ocular appearance guide treatment. A vitrectomy is both diagnostic and therapeutic but needs to take the overall clinical picture into consideration. A vitreous tap, and even more so an aqueous tap, is rarely useful when dealing with fungi, though polymerase chain reaction (PCR) can yield results when dealing with the more common fungi such as *Candida* and *Aspergillus* though its exact role in guiding treatment is yet to be determined.

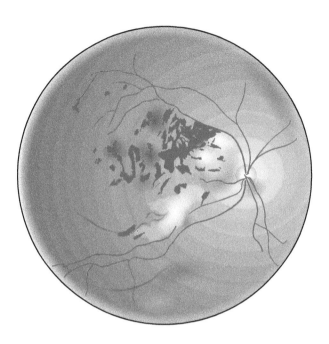

Figure 6.3 Ocular aspergillosis.

PANUVEITIS NOT DUE TO INFECTIOUS ENDOPHTHALMITIS WITH LOSS OF THE FUNDAL VIEW

This is a true diagnostic challenge as all the usual clues that help us are now removed. This situation is usually unilateral and a logical approach makes all the difference.

General management strategies – In all cases perform a B-scan ultrasound. This will assess the state of the retina and occasionally identify other potential diagnostic features such as a vitreous or vitreo-retinal abscess, a tumour such as a choroidal melanoma or retained lens matter. A vitreous tap should then be undertaken as described above with PCR sent for cytomegalovirus (CMV), herpes simplex virus (HSV), varicella zoster virus (VZV) and toxo-plasmosis, as well as bacterial and fungal culture and sensitivity. The laboratory should be contacted beforehand so you know how they want the samples and to alert them about their imminent arrival. Blood tests should include erythrocyte sedimentation rate (ESR), C-reactive protein (CRP), syphilis serology, toxoplasma IgG and IgM, full blood count (FBC) and urea and electrolytes (U and E). Have a low threshold for performing a HIV test.

Specific clinical presentations – In acute-onset panuveitis with no retinal view let us look at the most likely diagnoses in the correct order:

1. Bacterial endophthalmitis. In nearly all cases there will be a suggestive history – either of eye surgery, trauma or sepsis. In rare cases of endogenous endophthalmitis no source of underlying infection is ever found as occasionally patients may have bacteremia that is so transient that it passes almost unnoticed. As an extraordinarily rare event, devastating Streptococcal exogenous endophthalmitis can occur in an eye with no predisposing cause; it is theoretically conceivable that this highly pathogenic organism can penetrate the cornea after some minor surface trauma.

2. Toxoplasmosis panuveitis. Hypopyon uveitis is very uncommon in toxoplasmosis but is reported. Do not treat for this unless there are other clues such as the classic 'headlight in the fog' with a patch of retinitis surrounding a retinal scar.
3. Malignancy. In this case a pseudohypopyon might be present in the setting of a 'white eye'. Diseases include primary intraocular lymphoma, myeloma, metastatic disease, choroidal melanoma and retinoblastoma. If strongly suspected then AC tap for cytology and consider a formal vitreous biopsy.
4. Inflammatory non-infective causes. Think of very severe HLA-B27 disease, Behçet's disease and idiopathic causes.
5. Acute retinal necrosis (ARN) is extremely unlikely **if there is hypopyon present** – the authors have never seen ARN present with hypopyon.

Suggested initial management – Unless there are strong reasons to suspect otherwise we suggest a standard vitreous 'tap and inject' with ceftazidime 2 mg in 0.1 mL to cover the gram-negative organisms and vancomycin 1 mg in 0.1 mL to cover the gram positives, though amikacin 0.4 mg in 0.1 mL is sometimes used as an alternative to ceftazidime.

Acute-onset panuveitis with no retinal view and no hypopyon is a particularly tough challenge. If there is a history of sepsis, recent eye surgery or penetrating trauma then treat as bacterial endophthalmitis as per above. If there is no history of the above consider the following features:

- Is there granulomatous or non-granulomatous AC inflammation? You will need to consider diagnosis of ARN, toxoplasmosis chorioretinitis with panuveitis, syphilis or idiopathic non-infectious disease.
- Look for additional clues – Is the intraocular pressure (IOP) elevated? Is there a past history of previous toxoplasma chorioretinitis? Are there retinal scars in the fellow eye? Use the indirect ophthalmoscope as you might just see a patch of retinitis through dense vitritis, near a scar. If so, then perform an AC and vitreous tap with PCR sent for CMV, HSV, VZV and toxoplasmosis, as well as bacterial and fungal culture and sensitivity and treat for toxoplasmosis. If there is still some doubt, cover with an injection of foscarnet 2.4 mg in 0.1 mL which will provide antiviral cover in case you have mistaken a case of ARN for toxoplasmosis.

If none of the above then best treat as ARN. More commonly non-granulomatous AC reaction is present although this can be granulomatous and is not useful clinically in distinguishing ARN from other causes. The IOP is usually normal. You may see a patch of retinitis through dense vitritis, but usually no scar. In this situation ARN is the most dangerous differential to miss and so **valaciclovir 2 g three times a day (tds)** is a good treatment to start, preferably combined with intravitreal foscarnet 2.4 mg in 0.1 mL if readily available. Additionally an anti-toxoplasmal agent of your choice such as **azithromycin 500 mg od** or septrin (co-trimoxazole) 960 mg bd can be employed while results of the tap are awaited to cover for toxoplasmosis and **40 mg of prednisolone**, along with 30 mg of lansoprazole, to cover every inflammatory disorder.

Any anterior uveitis can be treated with topical Maxidex (dexamethasone) hourly along with a cycloplegic in the form of cyclopentolate 1% bd. As the picture improves and the results of the investigations come back then the unnecessary medications can be stopped. The first follow-up at 48 hours will be principally to review the microbiology results of cultures and to ensure the clinical picture is not drastically worse. The real results that guide treatment are the vitreous tap PCR results, which usually take 3–5 days. If any virus is shown on PCR then continue valaciclovir and consider a further intravitreal foscarnet injection. The steroids and the anti-toxoplasmal agent should be stopped completely and immediately. If the toxoplasmosis PCR is positive then the valaciclovir can be stopped and the anti-toxoplasmal antimicrobial continued along with a tapering dose of the steroid. The culture and sensitivity in these circumstances is rarely positive but if so the infectious endophthalmitis advice above should be followed. If the vitreous tap revealed nothing then the blood tests guide treatment.

Remember that syphilis can mimic all of the above, so all patients of sexually active age should have syphilis serology. Patients may deny high-risk activities so do not rely on the history. If the syphilis serology is positive a referral to the genitourinary clinic should immediately be made for penicillin treatment as detailed in the previous chapter. The antiviral and the anti-toxoplasmal agent can then be stopped and the steroids tapered by 10 mg per week. If the syphilis serology, the bacterial culture and viral PCR are all negative, but the toxoplasmosis serology is positive then the antiviral should be stopped and the advice in the toxoplasmosis section of the previous chapter followed.

If all of these tests are negative but the ESR and the CRP are high then an inflammatory disorder is likely and the valaciclovir and anti-toxoplasmal treatment can be discontinued. Continue oral steroids, topical steroids and cycloplegics. The patient can then be monitored on a weekly basis to await clearance of the vitreous. It is prudent to remember here that an indirect ophthalmoscope can reveal more details of the peripheral retina in a dense vitritis than any lens at the slit lamp and all effort should be made to obtain any view of any retina available. If the vitritis does not clear despite medication and time, then a vitreoretinal referral for a diagnostic vitrectomy should be made. This has two benefits. First, it will yield plenty of sample for bacterial and fungal culture, herpes viral PCR and Toxo PCR. You must send a sample also for cytology and histopathology as malignancy must be considered. Second, a diagnostic vitrectomy will allow you to view the retina.

An alternative and oft-missed condition that can mimic a posterior uveitis is lymphoma. It would be a less common presentation for it to present as a panuveitis but certainly if the vitreous tap is negative and the blood tests do not reveal any clue as to the cause and certainly if any treatment has no good effect beyond a mild transient improvement it should be considered. Always consider other malignant disorders – in children retinoblastoma and in adults choroidal melanoma, leukaemia, myeloma and metastatic disease.

Drug-induced causes – A full and detailed drug history should be taken as there are some medications that can cause a drug-induced uveitis. The anti-TB drug rifabutin in particular can cause a very severe panuveitis. As a general rule the more exotic sounding and rare the drug the more likely it is to cause uveitis, though a search should be made for any unusual drugs in the British National Formulary. There is no shame in Googling the names of the medications and some of the most renowned uveitis specialists in the world are not ashamed to look things up on Google. Asking a pharmacist for advice may also be useful though the best pharmacist in the world knows infinitely less than Google.

Sterile endophthalmitis from retained lens matter – These patients can present days or weeks after phacoemulsification cataract surgery. It is caused by an intense inflammatory reaction to retained lens matter, a 'dropped nucleus' arising as a result of complicated surgery. This causes a panuveitis, usually with marked elevation of IOP. Surgery may have been performed elsewhere and surgeons do not always own up this complication in the notes. First treat these patients as potentially post-operative infective cases with 'tap and inject'. Negative cultures will follow. The B-scan will show retained lens matter. Initial treatment is with intensive steroid therapy, both topical and systemic, in order to settle the inflammation, followed by vitrectomy to clear retained lens matter.

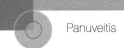
PRIMARY INTRAOCULAR LYMPHOMA

A lymphoma is a tumour that notoriously mimics various forms of uveitis and is very commonly missed for a variable length of time until the penny finally drops and somebody considers it. Of the myriad different presentations it is a variant of primary central nervous system (CNS) lymphoma which affects the eye, termed primary intraocular lymphoma (PIOL), that can fox the ophthalmologist. Of those with brain involvement 20% will develop eye involvement whereas of those presenting with ocular involvement alone 80% will go on to involve the brain. If the eyes are affected, 80% will be bilateral although there can be marked asymmetry and there may be months or years between onset of disease in the first and second eye. The typical patient is a woman in her 50s or 60s who develops a 'late-onset' uveitis. Typically the uveitis appears to be intermediate type, with 'vitritis', and is often misdiagnosed as such. A big trap is that, for a time, the uveitis appears to respond to steroids, at least initially, but after a while it worsens relentlessly. Uveitis presenting for the first time in later life should always be treated with suspicion.

Primary intraocular lymphoma presents with floaters and blur but rarely pain or photophobia. Examination will reveal cells and debris in the vitreous and possibly even what appears to be an anterior uveitis with keratic precipitates. So far so generic, but there are features that stand out, quite apart from the history, that point towards this diagnosis. The main feature is patches of subretinal tumour infiltration which are poorly defined yellow spots, dots or plaques, single or multiple, which appear under the retina (Figure 6.4). Other features include sheets of vitreous cells, the nature of which will raise suspicion of atypical vitritis, and an entirely white eye in the presence of significant anterior chamber cells. Otherwise PIOL can mimic any condition as cells leaving blood vessels can look like sheathing, occlusion of peripheral vessels can

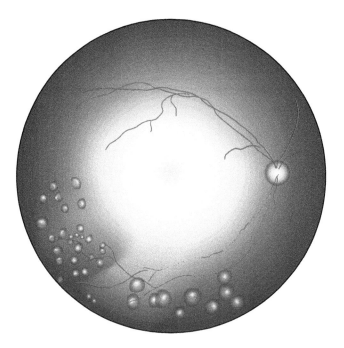

Figure 6.4 Subretinal infiltrates in primary intraocular lymphoma.

cause retinal necrosis, and cells in the anterior chamber can even form a hypopyon. Despite the presence of the above signs, cystoid macular oedema is quite rare (<3%) and the absence of CMO should raise suspicion. Finally, always think of this condition if the acuity is disproportionately worse or better than the clinical signs might suggest.

Tip: **Always consider this diagnosis when a person in their 50s or 60s presents with uveitis for the first time. Be especially aware of misdiagnosing this as intermediate uveitis.**

Should an older patient present with a panuveitis, typical or not, it is essential to ask about neurological symptoms such as balance issues, cognitive impairment, palsies, seizures and dizziness. Should PIOL be suspected you will need to order a brain and orbit magnetic resonance imaging (MRI) with contrast to look for intracranial involvement. A computed tomography (CT) brain scan is not an alternative to MRI, as although it might detect intracranial involvement in some, the sensitivity is not really good enough and it will miss disease. MRI should be performed within 6 weeks if there are no neurological symptoms and within a day or two if there are, with any abnormality suggestive of brain involvement prompting an immediate referral to the neurologists if possible, but if not the physicians, who can then liaise with the oncology team about treatment. Because primary CNS lymphoma is both life and sight threatening, and the implications are devastating, we have a duty as ophthalmologists to diagnose it promptly.

From an ophthalmic perspective an optical coherence tomography (OCT) scan can reveal infiltrates under the RPE – these are often discrete dome-like lesions and are highly suggestive of lymphoma. Fluorescein angiography demonstrates damage to the RPE through window defects and masking defects and in some this can result in a striking appearance which is termed the 'leopard spot angiogram'. The primary aim of all other investigations is to rule out other diagnoses that might be mimicked by the disease. Should no abnormality be found on the MRI scan but lymphoma still be suspected a diagnostic vitrectomy is the next step, though it is recommended that the patient should be sent to the nearest ocular oncology centre for this intervention to be carried out. This is because the pathology service in almost every other centre is not up to the task of processing the sample adequately, and transporting the sample elsewhere following a vitrectomy in the base hospital lowers the diagnostic yield. Even with a vitrectomy performed in an ocular oncology centre with excellent pathology the yield is low and it is not uncommon to have to perform several procedures separated by months before a positive sample is obtained. There is absolutely no point whatsoever in performing a clean room vitreous biopsy with a needle, other than to rule out other diagnoses if suspected. Certain studies have demonstrated that measuring the concentration of interleukin 10 (IL10) in the aqueous fluid or vitreous can aid diagnosis. This can be combined with measuring the ratio of interleukin 10 to interleukin 6 (IL10:IL6 ratio) which appears high in the majority of patients with PIOL.

Treatment is organised via the oncologists and has traditionally consisted of chemotherapy, with or without whole brain radiotherapy. There is recent interest in high-dose chemotherapy with autologous stem cell implant. Our role as ophthalmologists is confined to measuring the response. Rarely intravitreal methotrexate can be given for PIOL if the usual treatment has not been successful though this should be in close co-operation with the oncology and the haematology teams. It must also be remembered that intravitreal treatment does not prolong life and is an adjunct to systemic treatment specifically for the aim of stabilising sight, not an alternative, even if there is no apparent brain involvement. The prognosis of primary CNS lymphoma is pretty bleak, with a median survival of between 2.5 and 5 years after diagnosis. Early detection is key and even then, the prognosis, though better, is still quite poor, with most patients still dying of the disease. Having a low index of suspicion in older people presenting with an atypical bilateral uveitis which only transiently responds to steroids is critical.

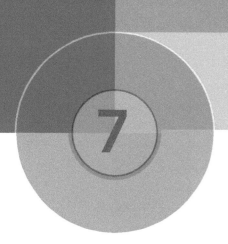

Scleritis and episcleritis

Scleritis is a condition that sits uneasily in the uveitis clinic. The sclera is not a part of the uveal tract and scleritis itself presents differently to uveitis and is treated differently. Uveitis trainees do not traditionally like such cases as they are out of the ordinary and require a different thought process, but in reality inflammation of the sclera is simple to understand and treatment follows a simple algorithm. The episclera is a thin layer of connective tissue that sits between the conjunctiva on the surface and the sclera beneath. Inflammation of this layer can present similarly but is treated differently to scleritis so knowing the difference is vital.

EPISCLERITIS

Every eye department in the world has a steady stream of worried young women presenting with a unilateral red eye that is diagnosed as episcleritis. The cause of this common condition is as yet unknown though the typical eye casualty spiel will tell how 'the immune system gets confused and starts attacking a layer of the eye' and when the patient asks why they are told 'not much is known but it might be a reaction to a virus or something'. The actual truth is even simpler though patients seldom want to hear that nobody knows anything about why their condition occurs. Patients typically present with a **unilateral** red eye which may be red in one sector of the bulbar surface, termed **sectoral**, or red all over, in which case it is **diffuse** (Figure 7.1). If the area of redness is flat the episcleritis is termed **simple** but if it is locally thickened it is called **nodular** (Figure 7.2). It may be entirely asymptomatic or cause a mild ache at most. The sclera by definition cannot be involved and the traditional eye casualty test involves putting a drop of phenylephrine 2.5% in the eye with complete resolution of the redness 10 minutes later confirming a diagnosis of episcleritis. When this wears off the redness will recur of course; this test is diagnostic not therapeutic. No further investigation is needed.

Most of the time no treatment is needed and simple reassurance will do as the natural course is for the condition to resolve spontaneously over a week or two in the case of simple episcleritis and 3–4 weeks with nodular episcleritis. Should the ache be problematic or more commonly the patient persistent, then ocular lubricants of any variety qds for 2 weeks can be prescribed. Should this not do the trick the next step up the ladder is a topical non-steroidal such as ketorolac tds for 2 weeks. The step above this is a weak topical steroid in the form of fluorometholone (FML) qds for 1 week followed by bd for 1 week. A stronger topical steroid in the form of Maxidex (dexamethasone 0.1%) following the same regime is the next step finally followed by oral non-steroidals such as flurbiprofen 100 mg tds for 2 weeks. Try to resist giving Maxidex as while it is

(a)

(b)

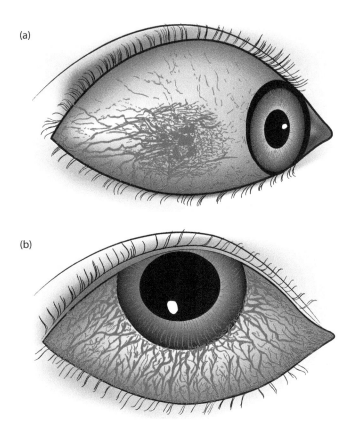

Figure 7.1 Sectoral and diffuse episcleritis.

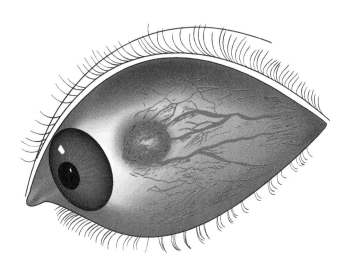

Figure 7.2 Nodular episcleritis.

indeed very effective, it should be avoided for the simple reason that the mildness of the condition does not justify the potential iatrogenic side effects of raised intraocular pressure and cataract acceleration. Considering the natural history, it might be thought that atypically long attacks or recurrent episodes would be needed to reach the top of the treatment algorithm but in practice the first step is to prescribe a lubricant and should the patient return they are given FML drops.

The main differential diagnosis is ocular surface disorder such as allergy, dry eye or contact lens related pathology and bilateral episcleritis should always arouse suspicion as it is so rare. Occasionally thyroid eye disease can be mistaken for episcleritis, but there will always be other signs of thyroid eye disease which should alert the clinician. The most important differential is of course scleritis but the mildness of the pain and the success of the phenylephrine test in blanching the redness should help differentiate one from the other.

SCLERITIS

Inflammation of the sclera itself is called scleritis. Scleritis is classified by location, with **anterior** affecting the sclera that can be seen and **posterior** affecting the sclera that cannot. Essentially if there is any redness that can be seen it is called anterior scleritis. It is further classified into **non-necrotising** and **necrotising** depending on whether the sclera becomes thinned and necrotic, which can be determined if the blue-black underlying choroid can be seen underneath or not. Non-necrotising anterior scleritis, as with episcleritis, is divided again into **diffuse** or **nodular**, although sectoral is not an option here. Necrotising anterior scleritis is said to occur **with inflammation** if the eye is red and painful or **without inflammation** if it is not. Table 7.1 better illustrates this confusing terminology.

Let us start with **non-necrotising anterior scleritis**. As with episcleritis it can be diffuse with redness all over or have a nodule in one place, commonly between the eyelids in the interpalpebral fissure. What differentiates it from episcleritis is the deep-seated pain that classically wakes a patient from their sleep, the tenderness of the globe itself and the long history. The pain is made worse by eye movements and while episcleritis affects young females scleritis tends to affect slightly older females. The clinical similarity with episcleritis might mean a patient goes many months with waxing and waning scleritis misdiagnosed as episcleritis with the very obvious tell-tale feature being the long history itself. A patient complaining 'I just can't shake this episcleritis' is a clear indication that the diagnosis should be questioned. The phenylephrine test mentioned above will likewise be positive in that application of drops will not clear up all the injection. Three-quarters of all scleritis cases fall into this category.

Patients often discover that the relentless pain can only be eased by large doses of oral non-steroidals such as ibuprofen. Distinguishing episcleritis from anterior diffuse scleritis can

Table 7.1 Classification of episcleritis and scleritis

Episcleritis	Simple	Sectoral
		Diffuse
	Nodular	
Scleritis	Non-necrotising	Diffuse
		Nodular
Anterior	Necrotising	With inflammation
		Without inflammation
Posterior – As anterior but can only be subclassified on B-scan ultrasound		

be tricky. Patients with scleritis always have very injected superficial vessels in the episcleral plexus, which is why misdiagnosis as episcleritis is such a common phenomenon. Careful inspection will reveal deep vessel engorgement and injection of the deeper scleral vessels. It is important to remember that a proportion of patients with anterior scleritis have associated posterior scleritis so have a low threshold for performing a B-scan in order to diagnose this.

Tip: **If episcleritis is persistent and does not clear quickly always consider scleritis.**

Unlike episcleritis half of all cases of scleritis are associated with a systemic disease and the most common disease is rheumatoid arthritis. Less common associations include granulomatosis with polyangiitis (formerly Wegener's disease), systemic vasculitis such as polyarteritis nodosa, relapsing polychondritis, systemic lupus erythematosus, spondylo-arthropathies and other auto-immune diseases. Infectious causes of scleritis are less common but include varicella zoster virus, syphilis and tuberculosis, which is very rare in the West but more common in endemic countries like India. Fungi, bacteria and acanthamoebae pathogens can cause a severe scleritis, usually in association with corneal infection. Finally, never forget that choroidal melanoma can sometimes cause a secondary adjacent inflammatory scleritis. It is always useful if a patient already has such a diagnosis but if not a careful history needs to be taken for joint issues, respiratory tract, nasal and sinus symptoms. Investigations should include **full blood count (FBC), urea and electro-lytes (U and E), erythrocyte sedimentation rate (ESR), C-reactive protein (CRP), rheuma-toid factor (RF), cyclic citrullinated peptide (CCP) antibody, syphilis serology** and **c-ANCA** (also known as PR3-ANCA). The other ANCA, p-ANCA, is associated with other conditions such as Churg-Strauss syndrome. CCP is another more accurate test for rheumatoid arthritis.

Even though lupus is a differential diagnosis ordering ds-DNA and antinuclear antibody (ANA) is not useful as these tests are so misleading and generally awful that no ophthalmologist should ever be ordering them. If there are joint issues regardless of the RF result a referral to a rheumatologist should be undertaken routinely. The ESR and CRP in this context will guide the rheumatologist as to the severity of the condition and how quickly they need to be seen. If there are respiratory tract symptoms and the c-ANCA is positive then granulomatosis with polyan-giitis should be suspected and the patient referred urgently to the rheumatology team, with a deranged U and E test on top of this mandating a same-day referral. If there is a high index of suspicion ask the patient to give a urine sample and perform a dipstick in the clinic as this will give an immediate result – the presence of blood and protein should result in an immediate phone call to the rheumatologists. If there are vague rheumatology symptoms and the blood tests are borderline it is best to refer to the rheumatologists and let them perform further investiga-tions rather than order anything extra ourselves. Rheumatology is its own specialty for a reason.

Managing non-necrotising anterior scleritis needs a consistent approach. In most cases it is sensible to commence therapy with the simplest agents first. If no response occurs therapy can be tailored and escalated to include more potent therapeutic agents. Oral non-steroidals in the form of flurbiprofen 100 mg tds is the best agent. Augment this with Maxidex (dexamethasone 0.1%) six times a day topically for 2 weeks. If the eye is improved then the flurbiprofen is tapered in stepwise fashion 100 mg bd for 2 weeks, 50 mg tds for 2 weeks, 50 mg bd for 2 weeks and 50 mg od for 2 weeks. Always add gastric protection, for example omeprazole 20 mg od. If the patient is intolerant try a COX-2 inhibitor like Meloxicam 15 mg once daily for 2 weeks and then reduce to 7.5 mg daily thereafter. Once the flurbiprofen is discontinued the topical Maxidex can be tapered as in anterior uveitis. If there is a good and prompt clinical response, then you can fol-low-up every 3 weeks, to ensure remission, and monitor the intraocular pressure. Monitor also for symptoms of non-steroidal anti-inflammatory drug (NSAID) side effects by asking about gastrointestinal intolerance and check renal function with U and E testing every 3–6 months.

If after 2 weeks no substantial improvement is observed with oral non-steroidals and Maxidex, therapy alteration should take place. There is little point in continuing with ineffective therapy. Switch to a course of oral steroids in the form of prednisolone 60 mg od tapering by 10 mg a week if bilateral disease is present, though if your patient has unilateral disease there are some other attractive options in the form of local steroids. Note that these must never be used if there is any suggestion of necrotising anterior scleritis, or infective scleritis. An orbital floor depot steroid of triamcinolone (Kenalog) 40 mg can work wonders. For more severe cases of anterior non-necrotising scleritis injecting **subconjunctival Kenalog** over the active areas can be used to achieve rapid control of severe non-necrotising scleritis. It is done in the following manner:

1. This injection can be done in the clinic room without needing a clean room. Shake the vial of Kenalog well.
2. Draw up 1 mL (40 mg) of Kenalog into a 1 mL syringe using a green needle (21 gauge). Using a filtered needle or a smaller needle will result in failure due to immediate blockage.
3. Swap the green needle for a short orange needle (25 gauge) and expel the air.
4. After instilling proxymetacaine in the conjunctival sac, place a cotton bud, soaked in Tetracaine against the area of active scleritis. Use several cotton buds if needed.
5. Instil topical phenylephrine – preferably 10%, over the injected area to help blanch the vessels.
6. Instil Povidone iodine 5% into the conjunctival sac.
7. Inject subconjunctival Kenalog. Aim to raise small blebs of between 0.05 and 0.2 mL of Kenalog, over the active areas of scleritis, but away from the limbus, usually giving one injection per quadrant.
8. Apply topical chloramphenicol at the end of the procedure.

Note that it is normal to cause some subconjunctival haemorrhage and the patient should be reassured that this will settle. Some patients may notice the subconjunctival Kenalog as an unsightly white lump but again this will resolve very slowly over 2–3 months and the patient needs to be reassured that this will not be a permanent feature.

Should the scleritis flare up after locally administered steroids, with or without NSAIDs then long-term corticosteroid therapy with or without steroid-sparing agents may be needed as described in Chapter 8. Our first choice of steroid-sparing agent for scleritis would be Methotrexate, as it works better for scleritis than Mycophenolate which is often ineffective. If that fails, Tacrolimus or Ciclosporin can be added. For resistant cases, biologicals should be considered. Anti-TNF agents such as Humira or Infliximab can be highly effective and if these agents fail to control the disease then consider Rituximab. Some specialists omit anti-TNF and go straight for Rituximab therapy. The authors have seen this drug induce remarkable remission in cases where all else has failed.

Necrotising anterior scleritis is differentiated from its non-necrotising cousin by the presence of an initial avascular patch or patches of sclera with central oedema. This becomes a thinned area with the blue hue of the underlying choroid showing through (Figure 7.3). This can be quite frighteningly large and quite hideously thinned and can perforate. Up to 60% of cases are bilateral and two thirds are with inflammation, a third without. In fact necrotising anterior scleritis without inflammation is a separate beast which will be dealt with later. The situation is more desperate than non-necrotising scleritis and thus while the investigations are the same the treatment should jump straight to the 60 mg of prednisolone stage. If perforation is a real danger referral to an anterior segment specialist is prudent for consideration of a scleral patch graft and some form of eye protection to avoid accidental injury in the meantime is advised.

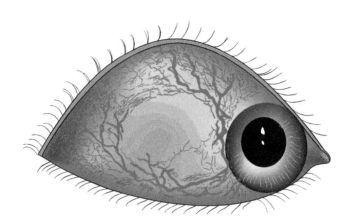

Figure 7.3 An area of scleral necrosis in a patient with necrotising anterior scleritis.

Necrotising anterior scleritis without inflammation is also known as scleromalacia perforans with the main difference being the complete lack of pain and the whiteness of the eye. Sometimes it is discovered incidentally where an oftentimes large and obvious black patch of clearly visible and protruding choroid in an otherwise white eye is discovered under the upper eyelid when the patient is asked to look down. Of the possible systemic diagnoses above rheumatoid arthritis is the condition overwhelmingly associated with this and history of joint disease is extremely common, for which a referral to a rheumatologist is advised. Investigations otherwise are identical to the non-necrotising variety above and treatment from an ophthalmic perspective is a lubricating eye drop six times a day in the affected eyes and prednisolone 60 mg tapering by 10 mg a week as detailed. Although actual perforation is rare referral to an anterior segment specialist and some form of eye protection to prevent accidental perforation is wise. Therapy for necrotising scleritis is similar, although rapid escalation to immunosuppressives and biologics is warranted.

Posterior scleritis is a different kettle of fish altogether. It may be associated with anterior scleritis as well in which case the treatment is the same and hence the posterior element may be missed altogether in all the excitement about the anterior component. When it occurs alone it can be difficult to diagnose as the eye is white and inflammation free on examination. Posterior scleritis is bilateral in less than 40% of cases and tends to occur in people less than 40 years old. The patient will present with severe pain in the eye described as a boring ache which is exacerbated by eye movement. The pain in fact appears totally out of proportion to the clinical signs which can be split into intraocular and extraocular manifestations. A thickened posterior sclera caused by inflammation may push the eye outward a small amount causing a mild proptosis, and as the extraocular muscles pass by the posterior sclera involvement of these can cause diplopia and is what is responsible for the painful eye movements. Note here however that if this feature is marked orbital myositis must first be considered the frontline diagnosis rather than a myositis secondary to a scleritis. Occasionally posterior scleritis can be entirely painless and this can catch the clinician out. Intraocular examination classically demonstrates choroidal folds and a swollen optic disc (Figure 7.4) with the more severe cases demonstrating an exudative retinal detachment. Sometimes sub-retinal masses can be identified. Peripheral choroidal annular effusions can induce secondary angle closure glaucoma.

The most useful clinical examination that can be performed in clinic is a B-scan ultrasound. This will demonstrate a thickening of the posterior coats of the eye, with a thickness greater than 2 mm considered abnormal. In unilateral disease a comparison can be made

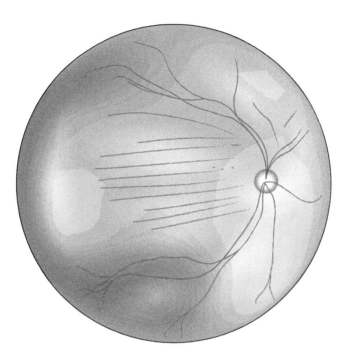

Figure 7.4 Fundal view of posterior scleritis.

with the unaffected eye. An additional textbook giveaway sign is fluid collecting between the sclera and Tenon capsule which results in the famous 'T sign' with the optic nerve and fluid forming the stem and arms of the letter 'T', respectively (Figure 7.5). The investigations for this are identical again to the above but on top of these, due to the different presentation other causes for choroidal folds and a swollen disc also need to be considered and ruled out, the most important of which is raised intracranial pressure. Other conditions that can mimic posterior scleritis include orbital inflammatory disease, choroidal haemangioma, uveal effusion syndrome, atypical central serous chorioretinopathy and Vogt–Koyanagi–Harada (VKH) syndrome. All of these will have distinctive features on fluorescein angiography, B-scan ultrasound (for instance the lack of a T sign), orbital and even brain MRI imaging that can help us distinguish between them.

As with anterior scleritis, posterior scleritis can present via either diffuse or nodular forms although this can only be appreciated on B-scan. Presumed necrotising posterior scleritis is very rare, but occasionally scleral thinning can be identified and these eyes can perforate, leading to sudden hypotony. About 30% of patients with posterior scleritis have an associated underlying systemic condition, with causes similar to those seen in anterior scleritis. In addition, lymphoma and myeloma have been reported as an extremely rare association.

The treatment algorithm is the same as for non-necrotising anterior scleritis above. It is worth mentioning that a peculiar feature of posterior scleritis is the persistence of pain even though the scleritis appears clinically inactive. Do not rely on pain as the sole indicator of activity, but instead use serial B-scans and the absence of the T sign as objective measures. The reason for this is that some patients appear to develop a chronic pain syndrome that causes discomfort even when the scleritis is inactive. In such cases, do not persist with oral steroids, immunosuppressives or biologicals, but steadily taper these agents. Patients with

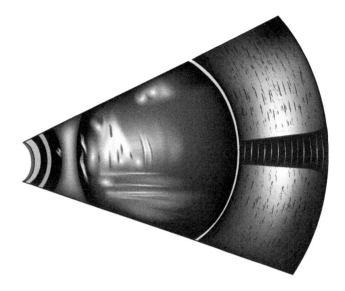

Figure 7.5 B-scan ultrasound demonstrating a 'T sign'.

persistent pain can benefit from agents like amitriptyline or gabapentin under the supervision of a pain clinic.

UVEAL EFFUSION SYNDROME

While uveal effusion syndrome is most certainly not a uveitic condition it is mentioned here as it can cause some diagnostic confusion, particularly in the case of posterior scleritis. In this condition a large collection of sub-retinal fluid develops, resulting in a serous, and often bullous, retinal detachment. This is accompanied by choroidal thickening. On examination chronic, spotty retinal pigment epithelial pigmentation develops, described as 'leopard spots', and are seen on fundus examination and are also visible on the FFA. The fluid build-up arises through an unknown mechanism which is thought in part to be due to an impaired scleral permeability preventing normal drainage. The patients often, but not always, have hypermetropic refraction and nanophthalmic eyes, so the patient's refraction and a measure of the axial length can be very useful in differentiating scleritis from uveal effusion syndrome. A lack of pain or inflammation can also help the clinician differentiate uveal effusion syndrome from posterior scleritis although as mentioned scleritis can, in some cases, also present without any pain at all. The treatment of the two is entirely different as in uveal effusion syndrome the altered scleral permeability of the abnormal sclera can be bypassed by performing a posterior partial thickness sclerectomy. Unlike scleritis oral steroids do not work, although given the rarity and difficulty of diagnosing this condition, many patients have accidentally been given steroids before uveal effusion syndrome is eventually diagnosed. This differentiation shows that medicine is an art as well as a science and that lateral thinking coupled with an enquiring mind can make all the difference.

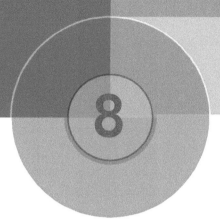

Immunosuppression: Medications, and how to use and monitor them

8

There are many detailed textbooks in existence about immunosuppression and whole tables and long, long lists about the side effects of the various medications. Indeed a common medical school exercise is to go around a group of students asking each one in turn to name a side effect of oral corticosteroid therapy and it is usual to be able to make several circuits before the group runs out of ideas. The true test however arises when it comes down to when and how to use these powerful medications. Nuclear physicists such as Otto Frisch and J. Robert Oppenheimer all had deep knowledge on how to construct, arm and detonate a nuclear bomb but hardly any about how to conduct a nuclear war. In reality it is knowledge about when and how to conduct a thermonuclear war that is essential to the survival of a nation and not so much the knowledge of the intricacies of the device.

What is not typically written in any traditional uveitis textbook is when to start various immunosuppressive agents and how to change doses when in fact this is the knowledge that ophthalmologists working in medical retina clinics up and down the land really need. Doctors faced with a patient on a specific dose of a specific medication; what needs to be done? In reality what is typically done is that the eye is examined and if it is deemed quiet the last few letters are quickly scanned to see if there has been any change in dosage and if not the doctor will look to see where the boss is. The boss will be examining a patient with another two or three people waiting to ask him about their own patients so with a sigh the ophthalmologist will simply copy what his predecessor has done by keeping the dose the same and reviewing in the same interval that his predecessor had chosen.

So first why start any medication? To make the eye quiet. Why do we want to do that? To save sight. How does keeping the eye quiet save sight? By preventing glaucoma, cataract, cystoid macular oedema and progression of any retinal disease. Every patient should ask these three questions but because they never do we forget the answers. When the eye becomes quiet we want to keep it quiet. There is simply not enough published evidence to know what we should do for sure so we fall back on common sense. There will be specific exceptions of course such as Fuchs heterochromic iridocyclitis in which the inflammation very rarely needs treatment or birdshot chorioretinopathy in which the inflammation can be very mild but needs treatment as it is relentless. Otherwise the aims will be as follows:

Aim 1: To make an inflamed eye quiet
Aim 2: After the eye is quiet to try and withdraw treatment
Aim 3: Should treatment be tapered or withdrawn and the eye become inflamed to again restart treatment but keep treated for longer before trying to withdraw again – 6 months

Aim 4: Should the eye again become inflamed keep treatment ongoing for 2 years before again attempting to withdraw treatment

Aim 5: While treatment is ongoing to find a balance between enough immunosuppression that keeps the eye quiet and the least toxic dose possible

These are five simple aims. It is easy to lose track when seeing a patient about the length of time they have been on treatment, whether a reduction in dose is needed or if simply staying the course is best. Always ask how long they have been on treatment, when the last flare-up was and what the plan is. It is simply not sufficient to see if the eye is quiet, keep the dose the same and carry on. Likewise it is not sufficient to go through endless cycles of putting the dose of immunosuppressant up if the eye is inflamed and down if it is not. The aims must always be clear and the simpler the aims the better. Exceptions notwithstanding the quick taper, 6 months, 2 years rule is a good one to follow (Table 8.1).

The agent used is dependent on the step. Initially the agent of choice is oral corticosteroid in the form of prednisolone, which is usually started at a dose of 60 mg though 1 mg/kg is also commonly stated. If the patient is not obviously obese then 60 mg is sufficient with weight-dependent dosing only needed if the patient looks as if 60 mg might not cut the mustard. There is simply no need to use higher doses if the patient is of normal weight as 80 mg, 100 mg or even higher doses do not have a dramatically better effect on the eye though the chances of necrosis of the femoral head and other horrible complications do increase. Oral corticosteroids are fast acting and are the first-line therapy for getting the situation under control. Local therapy in the form of drops or injections are covered in the relevant chapters though as a general rule with posterior or panuveitis these are only used during episodes of flare-up and play little role in long-term maintenance. The disease by definition is systemic and we are treating the immune system not the isolated effect on the eyes. A rapid taper mechanism is displayed in Table 8.2.

Traditionally decisions are made at the 10 mg dose phase unless the eye flares up at a higher dose. If that does indeed happen, say at the 15 mg level, then the regime is restarted but at the level above that reached when the flare-up occurred, in this case the 20 mg stage, the tapering is slowed down and the 1 week steps may be stretched to 2 weeks or longer. Intermediate stages can also be added of 15 mg/10 mg alternate days, for example, but the aim of this is to finish a

Table 8.1 The three steps of immunosuppressive therapy

Step	Duration of immunosuppression
Step 1	Once the eye is quiet attempt rapid taper
Step 2	Once the eye is quiet taper after 6 months
Step 3	Once the eye is quiet taper after 2 years

Table 8.2 A rapid taper oral corticosteroid regimen

Dose of oral prednisolone (mg)	Duration
60	1 week
40	1 week
30	1 week
20	1 week
15	1 week
10	1 week
5	1 week

rapid taper within 3 months. It is a testing of the enemy. There are only two outcomes: either the eye is tamed or it is not. If it is not then the second step needs to be implemented and this needs the eye to be quietened first and again corticosteroids in the form of oral prednisolone are the best for achieving rapid results. This time a 'steroid-sparing agent' will be started at the same time, provided the blood results are stable, and the steroid tapered to the dose above where the flare-up occurred last time.

Let us say the flare-up occurred when the dose fell to lower than 20 mg of prednisolone when the rapid taper was attempted, during step 2 the weaning of the prednisolone will take place until 20 mg is reached in the same manner as before and then arrested. It will be arrested until the steroid-sparing agent has reached its effective dose and has been given enough time to work and then the prednisolone will again be slowly tapered until a safe dose is reached. Although controversial, the safe dose is accepted by most authorities to lie at 7.5 mg a day. Once this is achieved there will be no further changes until 6 months have passed and then tapering can once again take place. The steroids are then tapered off completely in the same sized steps as with the rapid tapering regime though over a longer time period. There is absolutely no sense in using 1 or 2 mg steps as these simply prolong the process for no good reason. After the steroid has been tapered to nothing, tapering of the steroid-sparing agent can begin. Table 8.3 displays a typical regime of steroids with an addition of a steroid-sparing agent. Let us say again for the sake of this example that the previous flare-up occurred at the 15 mg level.

If this process is completed and the eye stays quiet the steroid-sparing agent is then tapered and stopped. If another flare-up occurs then the process is repeated but instead of 6 months the eye is kept quiet for 2 years before further tapering can take place. The aim of the steroid-sparing agent is to enable the magical dose of 7.5 mg of prednisolone to be reached but should this not be possible due to reactivation of the uveitis, despite another agent, four questions need to be asked:

Question 1: Is the patient fully compliant with the medication?
Question 2: Is the steroid-sparing agent at the highest end of the therapeutic range or can it be further increased?
Question 3: Can another agent be added?
Question 4: Is it time for a biologic agent?

Table 8.3 Prednisolone regime with a steroid-sparing agent added

Dose of oral prednisolone	Duration
60 mg	1 week
40 mg	1 week
30 mg	1 week
20 mg	Until steroid-sparing agent effective
15 mg/20 mg alternate days	2 weeks
15 mg	2 weeks
10 mg/15 mg alternate days	2 weeks
10 mg	4 weeks
5 mg/10 mg alternate days or 7.5 mg	Until 6 months from start point reached
5 mg	4 weeks
0 mg/5 mg alternate days or 2.5 mg	4 weeks

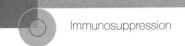

Let us look at each agent in turn, beginning with prednisolone. This is far from an exhaustive guide and only the most important features of each medication will be discussed. **How** to use the medication is paramount here.

PREDNISOLONE

This wonder drug has been mentioned numerous times throughout the book so far and the side-effect profile is both large and alarming. Table 8.4 gives a rundown of the potential side effects and how to avoid them.

There are legion side effects of course beyond these which may be of lesser significance to us but much more so for the patient. Weight gain, acne and sleep disturbance can affect the patient greatly and add to an emotional strain already at breaking point due to the direct effect of the medication. Steroid **psychosis** and **violent mood swings** are a very real phenomenon and this, more than any of the other potential side effects, can take the ophthalmologist out of their comfort zone faster than and more comprehensively than may at first be appreciated. Between them the authors have come across a normally quiet and respectable man come close to punching his wife in the clinic out of sheer anger after high-dose oral steroid commencement, as well as an elderly patient being admitted temporarily under a section of the mental health act for attempting to climb a lamppost in the street outside the hospital in the erroneous belief that her very life depended on it. Therefore, should a patient mention that they feel strange, aggressive, depressed or psychotic do not simply offer a reassuring smile as you lead them to the door but **take these concerns very seriously** and be prepared to act on them by reducing the dose or indeed stopping it altogether. More commonly, many patients on long-term steroids report a less dramatic but profoundly debilitating dampening of their mood. Others report sleep disturbance as an overwhelmingly prominent symptom.

Other side effects with which we need to be concerned include hypertension, skin thinning and bruising, fluid retention and hyperlipidaemia. Patients with pre-existing obesity, diabetes, osteoporosis, infection or psychiatric disease need to be treated with caution when contemplating the commencement of steroid therapy and warned of all the potential side effects that apply to them in particular.

Before starting steroid therapy it is essential to check both blood pressure and blood sugar (BM), both of which can be done in the eye clinic. After starting it is prudent to ask the general practitioner (GP) to monitor BM, lipids and arrange dual-energy x-ray absorptiometry (DEXA) scanning though in very large uveitis units this can be arranged in-house. A dedicated system of uveitis nurses to organise tests and to follow up the results is ideal although in practice

Table 8.4 Prednisolone side effects and monitoring

Side effect	Monitoring/treatment
Diabetes or if diabetic worsening control	Blood sugar (BM)
Weight gain and hyperlipidaemia	Serum lipid testing
Peptic ulceration	Co-prescription of **30 mg of lansoprazole**
Osteoporosis	Co-prescription of **Calcichew two tablets once a day** and yearly DEXA scan
Cataract	Examination at slit lamp
Ocular hypertension	Goldman tonometry

most units do not have this luxury and the GP is a more well-rounded clinician, better able to monitor these things. Traditionally uveitis specialists are notoriously forgetful when it comes to things outside of the eye and it is not unusual for patients to go years without a DEXA scan if ophthalmologists alone are responsible for monitoring this. A good working relationship with a GP is vital and some general practitioners are so hands on that they will prescribe the medication out of their own budget and perform all of the monitoring bloods for the steroid-sparing agents, though before relying on this it is of course essential that it is checked, lest the patient fall between two stools. Some units have specific letters for each medication started including prednisolone that are sent to patients' GPs with clear boundaries about who takes care of what. Despite this the shared care arrangements are the most problematic arrangement in uveitis clinics and all further tables will be arranged as if all medication is prescribed and dosed by the ophthalmologists and all blood testing and monitoring is done likewise. DEXA scanning is a special case, as is diabetic control and lipid control as these are the traditional remit of the GP in Wales and most of the rest of the United Kingdom.

When started on long-term oral steroid treatment, and by extension all immunosuppressive agents, the patient should be assessed for the possibility of previous tuberculosis (TB) and asked if they have previously had varicella zoster infection (chickenpox or shingles). If there is a possibility of TB then testing may need to be done to avoid a life-threatening flare-up later on. If there is no history of varicella zoster virus exposure such as chickenpox or shingles, serology looking for previous asymptomatic infection should be undertaken. As the vaccine takes too long to work for delaying the start of immunosuppression to be feasible in almost all of the situations encountered in this book, the patient should be warned to keep away from those with active infection of either chickenpox or shingles, and told all about the symptoms of infection so that it can be reported immediately should it occur. Treatment with oral acyclovir 800 mg five times a day for 2 weeks at least is then required with discontinuation of immunosuppression should the situation get out of hand. In heavily immunosuppressed patients intramuscular varicella zoster immunoglobulin may be required but this is the domain of the physicians and our role is simply to get the patient to the right physician as quickly as possible and to be alert to the possibility of this happening. The vaccine is a live vaccine so cannot be given once immunosuppression has started. This is the reason why all vaccinations should be checked in immunosuppressed patients to ensure they are safe. With steroids the possibility of an Addisonian crisis should the patient suddenly stop their medication must also be explained, though in reality this seems rare.

Tip: Check to see if it is safe to administer a vaccine, if required, in an immunosuppressed patient.

INTRAVENOUS METHYLPREDNISOLONE

There are instances where even more rapid control of the inflammation is required for reasons specific to each disease in which case **intravenous methylprednisolone** 1 g once a day for 3 days is the standard treatment. It is mixed with normal saline and administered over a 30-minute duration. It is a bit of a nuclear option and as such patients with active infection, cardiac failure, uncontrolled diabetes and psychosis or other mood disturbances should not be given this powerful medication. Nursing staff monitor blood pressure (BP), BM and pulse rate half hourly for the duration of the infusion and for an hour afterwards. If during the infusion the blood pressure rises to above 100 mmHg diastolic it should be immediately stopped. The infusion of methylprednisolone is done as an inpatient in most units due to the sheer organisation required in a National Health System (NHS) setting, though if there is a day facility whereby this can take place that would be preferable to occupying an inpatient bed. The considerations are all the same as for oral prednisolone except that the potential problems can be even worse. Other side effects such as a temporary psychosis become more common with intravenous steroid treatment and chest pain or even cardiovascular collapse can occur during the infusion which is why close monitoring is so essential. It should be noted, however, that some of the other side effects associated with oral steroid use, notably the Cushingoid appearance, are less common with intravenous administration.

STEROID-SPARING AGENTS

These agents can be split into three groups: The anti-metabolites, the calcineurin inhibitors and other cytotoxic agents that are too scary for an ophthalmologist to consider using. Agents in this last group include **chlorambucil**, derived from the mustard gas used in the trenches of the First World War, and **cyclophosphamide**, a slightly less toxic alternative that is still hideously toxic. These are dangerous medications that only a highly selective group of specialists use and they will not be mentioned here again. Table 8.5 shows which commonly used mediations are in which category.

It is important to know these groups as if needed two agents can be used together but *never* **two agents from the same group, or the patient might die**. That is the serious nature of these medications. There are various brand names for these medications and even though the active ingredient is the same and the dose the same they are not interchangeable for complicated pharmacological reasons and once started on one brand a patient should be kept on that brand. The side effects of all these medications are difficult to remember separately so the main ones are displayed in Table 8.6.

Table 8.5 Classes of steroid-sparing agents and the time it takes for them to become effective

Anti-metabolites	Time to action	Calcineurin inhibitors	Time to action
Mycophenolate mofetil	1 month	Tacrolimus	3 weeks
Methotrexate	3 months	Ciclosporin	2 weeks
Azathioprine	1 month		

Table 8.6 Main side effects of all the major steroid-sparing agents

Drug	Bone marrow	Liver	Kidneys	Other
Mycophenolate mofetil	Yes	Yes	Yes	Gastrointestinal disturbances
Methotrexate	Yes	Yes	Yes	Gastrointestinal disturbances
Azathioprine	Yes	Yes	No	Gastrointestinal disturbances
Tacrolimus	No	Yes	Yes	Hypertension Neurotoxicity
Cyclosporin	No	Yes	Yes	Hypertension Gum hyperplasia

Rather than remember each one separately it is better to think that bone marrow suppression, hepatotoxicity and nephrotoxicity are common to all and gastrointestinal disturbances and hypertension to some, with some extra specific ones thrown in for good measure.

PREGNANCY AND TERATOGENICITY

While oral steroids are thought to be mostly safe in pregnancy, other than an association between high doses and prolonged courses with intrauterine growth restriction, it is a different matter with steroid-sparing agents. This is particularly relevant to the patients who attend uveitis clinics as they tend to be younger than those attending general eye clinics and of child-bearing age. As a general rule females need two clear pregnancy tests prior to commencing steroid-sparing immunosuppressants and should they be sexually active after commencement, they must employ **two** different modes of contraception simultaneously to reduce the risk of pregnancy as much as possible. It is recommended that males on immunosuppressant medication also employ contraception though there is no convincing evidence of increased risk to any pregnancy that may result.

Although it is recommended that all immunosuppressants are avoided in pregnancy some are in fact safer than others. Methotrexate and mycophenolate mofetil should both be avoided absolutely as the risks of teratogenicity in both are very clear. Azathioprine and ciclosporin are both associated with increased rates of low birth weight and spontaneous abortion but otherwise can cautiously be considered safe. There is limited evidence, however tacrolimus needs to be treated with more caution in pregnancy due to teratogenicity in animal studies, but it is not absolutely contraindicated as with methotrexate and mycophenolate. For males, again there is much less data available, but it might be considered sensible to follow the same advice as for females. Anti-TNF agents (see Chapter 9) are considered safe in pregnancy for both men and women.

MYCOPHENOLATE MOFETIL

This agent is the most common steroid-sparing agent used. It works reasonably quickly in a few weeks with an acceptable side-effect profile with most patients tolerating it with little problem. Table 8.7 indicates how it is started and the dose increased while Table 8.8 indicates the monitoring schedule. The shaded boxes indicate the therapeutic range within which the dose should only be increased if further immunosuppression is required. If the dose is increased the monitoring schedule should return to baseline again. Tests to perform prior to starting the medication include **blood pressure (BP), weight, full blood count (FBC), urea and electrolytes (U and E), liver function test (LFT)** and **glucose**.

It can be seen that after a year and 3 months all the tests are performed every 2 months (8 weekly). It is important to keep a record of where the patient is in the schedule as it is very easy to get lost, though in fact the greatest sin is performing too many blood tests rather than too

Table 8.7 Mycophenolate mofetil dosing

Dose	Duration
Start – 500 mg bd	2 weeks
1 g bd	6 weeks
1 g am 1.5 g pm	6 weeks
1.5 g bd	Maximum dose

Table 8.8 Mycophenolate mofetil monitoring

Weeks after dose change	1	2	3	4	6	8	10	12	Beyond 12 weeks
FBC	Yes	Yes	Yes	Yes	Yes	Yes	Yes	Yes	Every month for a year then every 2 months
U and E					Yes			Yes	Every 2 months
LFT					Yes			Yes	Every 2 months
Glucose					Yes			Yes	Every 2 months

few as it is quicker and lazier to tick all the boxes than work out precisely where the patient is on the schedule. Should a swap of steroid-sparing agent be required a washout period identical to that in Table 8.5 must be observed prior to starting another agent.

METHOTREXATE

Methotrexate is slightly easier to manage than mycophenolate as the dosing is once a week and therefore ideal for children and those reluctant to take daily medication. The monitoring schedule is simple and easy to follow compared with other medications. On the downside this drug takes a relatively long time to start working on the immune system and is weaker than the others. Another downside is that weekly folic acid needs to be taken on a different day to the methotrexate, classically 3 days later, which can cause confusion. Table 8.9 indicates how it is started and the dose increased while Table 8.10 indicates the monitoring schedule. The shaded boxes indicate that the drug is started within its therapeutic range and the dose should only be increased if further immunosuppression is required. If the dose is increased the monitoring schedule should return to baseline again. Tests to perform prior to starting the medication include **FBC, U and E** and **LFT**.

Table 8.9 Methotrexate dosing

Dose	Duration
Start – 12.5 mg a week (+5 mg folic acid 3/7 later)	6 weeks
15 mg a week (+5 mg folic acid 3/7 later)	6 weeks
17.5 mg a week (+5 mg folic acid 3/7 later)	6 weeks
20 mg a week (+5 mg folic acid 3/7 later)	6 weeks
22.5 mg a week (+5 mg folic acid 3/7 later)	6 weeks
25 mg a week (+5 mg folic acid 3/7 later)	Maximum dose

Table 8.10 Methotrexate monitoring

Weeks after dose change	2	4	8	Beyond 8 weeks
FBC	Yes	Yes	Yes	Every 2 months
U and E	Yes	Yes	Yes	Every 2 months
LFT	Yes	Yes	Yes	Every 2 months

Table 8.11 Azathioprine dosing

Dose	Duration
Start – 50 mg bd	6 weeks
75 mg bd	6 weeks
100 mg bd	Maximum dose

AZATHIOPRINE

Azathioprine has a slightly more complicated monitoring protocol and prior to starting it a special test needs to be done for thiopurine methyltransferase (TPMT) levels. This should be above 67 mU/L as to cut a long story short this enzyme metabolises azathioprine and if the levels are low you might end up giving the equivalent of a lethal dose of azathioprine. If the levels are very low azathioprine should be avoided altogether but if above 20 mU/L it can still be given though cautiously and at a much reduced dose. In this instance halving all the doses stated below is best. Table 8.11 indicates how it is started and the dose increased while Table 8.12 indicates the monitoring schedule. The shaded boxes indicate the therapeutic range of the drug and the dose should only be increased if more immunosuppression is required. If the dose is increased the monitoring schedule should return to baseline again. Tests to perform prior to starting the medication include **TPMT, FBC, U and E, LFT, glucose** and **BP**. It is also vital to check if the patient is taking allopurinol, a common drug given for gout, as this produces an effect similar to a TPMT deficiency and the azathioprine dose is then reduced to a quarter of what it otherwise would be, or an alternative immunosuppressant considered.

TACROLIMUS

This drug is generally well tolerated though as with all these medications has a long list of potential side effects, including hypertension, hepatic dysfunction, gastrointestinal disturbance and interestingly the potential for both alopecia and hirsutism. Tacrolimus often causes a fine resting tremor, which is most noticeable in the hands. Tacrolimus is a trickier drug to control due to the need to monitor so called 'trough' levels. These are meant to indicate the level of a drug 12 hours after it is taken and for a twice-a-day drug like tacrolimus this means essentially right at the point before a tablet is taken but not after. Patients tend to take their medication at 8 a.m. and 8 p.m., neither of which are great times for blood samples. On top of this patients get terribly confused about this trough level and might take their tablet anyway 'as it was past time' thus giving a horribly elevated result which will result in unnecessary dose reduction. Either that or patients suspend their medication in the erroneous belief that this is what trough means, resulting in an undetectably low level and thus dangerous dose increases. The aim is to get the trough level stable at 5–10 micrograms/L though in reality the sensitivity of this to timing and patient fallibility means that all results should be taken with a pinch of

Table 8.12 Azathioprine monitoring

Weeks after dose change	1	2	3	4	8	12	16	Beyond 16 weeks
FBC	Yes	Yes	Yes	Yes	Yes		Yes	Every 2 months
U and E				Yes	Yes	Yes	Yes	Every 2 months
LFT				Yes	Yes	Yes	Yes	Every 2 months

Table 8.13 Tacrolimus dosing

Dose	Duration
Start – 1 mg bd	4 weeks
2 mg a.m.; 1 mg p.m.	4 weeks
2 mg bd	4 weeks
3 mg a.m.; 2 mg p.m.	4 weeks
3 mg bd	Maximum dose

Table 8.14 Tacrolimus monitoring

Weeks after dose change	2	4	6	8	10	12	Beyond 12 weeks
FBC	Yes	Yes		Yes		Yes	Every 2 months
U and E	Yes	Yes	Yes	Yes	Yes	Yes	Every month/4 weeks
LFT	Yes	Yes		Yes		Yes	Every 2 months
Tacrolimus trough level	Yes	Yes		Yes		Yes	Every 2 months
Glucose		Yes		Yes		Yes	Every 2 months
Blood pressure		Yes		Yes		Yes	Every 2 months
Lipid and magnesium						Yes	Every 6 months

salt. Table 8.13 indicates how it is started and the dose increased while Table 8.14 indicates the monitoring schedule. There are no coloured boxes this time as it is the trough level that determines whether the drug has reached its therapeutic range. If the dose is increased the monitoring schedule should return to baseline again. Tests to perform prior to starting the medication include **FBC, U and E, LFT, glucose, BP** and **weight**.

As Table 8.13 suggests start at 1 mg bd and immediately prior to increasing the dose obtain a trough level. Trough levels should be obtained prior to all dose changes whether it fits in with the schedule in Table 8.14 or not. In most, but not all patients, the initial trough level will be very low, but tacrolimus is strange in that some patients need only a small dose while others need a lot more to obtain the same trough levels. The reason for this is not properly understood but it is thought to be related to poor absorption. Also note that while the vast majority of patients need not be on any more than the range in Table 8.13 a small minority may need up to 4 mg twice daily (bd) but as this is tricky to manage and could potentially cause harm we have excluded these last high-dose steps from the protocol. The same absorption issue is thought to be responsible.

CICLOSPORIN

Ciclosporin, also called cyclosporine or cyclosporin A, is regarded as the slightly nastier brother of tacrolimus that is more aggressive in doing the job but nastier as it goes about it. Interestingly it is an antibiotic that was derived from experimenting on soil from Easter Island where the population was efficient in producing hundreds upon hundreds of carved heads though their aggressive nature and devastating interaction with the environment and with each other led to their near extinction is a sobering microcosm of humanity's tenuous hold on Planet Earth. The side-effect profile is similar to tacrolimus, but worse. It is therefore much more likely to cause renal impairment than tacrolimus and this is a major problem with prolonged use. There are added side effects such as gingival hyperplasia, hirsutism, a painful peripheral neuropathy

Table 8.15 Ciclosporin dosing

Dose	Duration
Start – 100 mg bd	4 weeks
150 mg bd	4 weeks
200 mg bd	Maximum dose

Table 8.16 Ciclosporin monitoring

Weeks after dose change	2	4	8	12	Beyond 12 weeks
FBC	Yes	Yes	Yes	Yes	Every 2 months
U and E	Yes	Yes	Yes	Yes	Every 2 months
LFT	Yes	Yes	Yes	Yes	Every 2 months
Glucose		Yes		Yes	Every 2 months
Blood pressure	Yes	Yes		Yes	Every 2 months
Lipid and magnesium				Yes	Every 6 months

and dental issues that need to be kept in mind. Though trough levels can be measured for ciclosporin they are currently utterly useless in the practical management of the disease as the therapeutic window overlaps with undetectably low trough levels. Table 8.15 indicates how it is started and the dose increased while Table 8.16 indicates the monitoring schedule. The shaded boxes indicate the therapeutic range of the drug and the dose should only be increased if more immunosuppression is required. If the dose is increased the monitoring schedule should return to baseline again. Tests to perform prior to starting the medication include **FBC, U and E, LFT, glucose, BP** and **weight**.

Please note that Table 8.15 is based on a person 70 kg in weight. The recommended doses are derived from this assumption but as ciclosporin is more sensitive to weight dosing than the other medication in this chapter it may be useful to bear in mind that the recommended first step is at 2.5 mg/kg, the following step 4 mg/kg and the top dose 5 mg/kg. The patient must be weighed and if they are significantly heavier or lighter than 70 kg the dose adjustments must follow this regimen.

The dose can be further increased but Table 8.15 specifically excludes higher doses as extreme caution needs to be taken above 200 mg bd and it is not for the fainthearted patient or ophthalmologist. Interestingly the lower starting dose of 100 mg bd may also be effective though only after higher doses have been used and the dose subsequently reduced. This whole area is controversial and different specialists will have their own protocol and reasoning.

Cyclosporin is one of the few drugs that should not be stopped suddenly, if it can be at all avoided. Unless there is an urgent need to stop the drug, such as sudden severe renal impairment, decrease the dose gradually in 50–100 mg decrements every 2 months. The reason for the gradual taper is that sudden cessation is associated with a severe rebound in inflammatory activity. The drug is unusual in this effect.

PRACTICAL ADVICE ON DRUG MONITORING

It can be seen that every regime is different and complicated and utterly impossible to remember. In addition to this different clinics do things differently so it is not consistent. The above represents a safe protocol that closely aligns with what most centres utilise in their uveitis service. In order to simplify things some centres use a piece of paper with all the monitoring intervals on which is filed into the patient's notes, others use a computer system and still others use a uveitis specialist nurse who co-ordinates all the visits, the blood tests and other monitoring essentials. Even so it is very common for patients to become lost on their monitoring schedules and for important blood tests to be missed and blood pressures forgotten. It is therefore critical that the clinical lead in the uveitis service and the consultant in clinic emphasise the importance of adhering to the monitoring protocol and for clear documentation in the notes to explain where the patient is on that schedule so that those seeing the patient in later visits know where they are and what they are supposed to do. It can be imagined that if care within a single hospital department is complicated, shared care with a general practitioner utilising a postal means of communication has the potential to result in great problems, so if a shared care model is adopted the ophthalmologist must be crystal clear in his own mind that the protocol is being followed. It is literally a matter of life or death.

The doses above are based on those commonly used in people of a normal weight of 70–80 kg. If the patient is a bit light or, as is much more common in this day and age, substantially heavier than what would be expected, dosing by weight is needed. Likewise a full drug history needs to be taken as well as the doses above also apply only to those not taking drugs which interact. Unlike patients in some other clinics those attending for uveitis are more likely to be young and female. For this reason advising against pregnancy is very important and may be one of the few occasions when ophthalmologists give advice on contraception.

'Making sure the bloods are okay' is also potentially more problematic than it seems. It is not simply a quick glance at the screen to see if any of the numbers are red and if not handing the patient another blood form and putting a tick next to the word 'bloods' in the notes. There are specific issues to consider, the most important of which is the FBC. Of this the most important parameters to watch are the **white cell count** (WCC) which cannot be allowed to fall below 3×10^9/L, the **neutrophils** which cannot be allowed to fall below 2×10^9/L and the **lymphocyte** count which cannot be allowed to fall below 0.6×10^9/L. The lymphocyte count is the most important of these as we *do* want there to be an effect on the immune system but not too much. If the lymphocyte count is blue on the screen and not red then we have to question what the therapy is actually achieving. The lower limit of normal for the lymphocyte count is 1×10^9/L and between 0.6 and 1×10^9/L is the sweet spot for which to aim. As with all aiming it should not be suddenly achieved and trajectory is as important if not more important than single results, and sudden achievement of the target should ring alarm bells. If immediately after commencing a medication the lymphocytes drop substantially to 0.8×10^9/L it is far more worrying than if after a dose increase the lymphocytes fall from 0.7×10^9/L to 0.6×10^9/L. Some authorities say that a rogue result of 0.5×10^9/L is acceptable while others would not. As with steering a ship it is important not to make any sudden and violent movements of the rudder as adjustments here take time to work their way through to a change of direction and persist after a readjustment has taken place.

It is important to ascertain when the patient is in danger and a sudden variation in a blood test parameter, especially coupled with the emergence of a new symptom, is potentially problematic. If the lymphocytes drop suddenly or any of the acceptable blood parameters above are passed then two options exist – to stay the course with a reduced dose or to stop the medication altogether until everything has recovered. This is an art, not a science, and knowing previous trends is vital to knowing what will likely transpire. Care must be taken at every step. Last it must be remembered that there is a patient behind the uveitis and to the uninitiated the disease and the therapy are confusing and frightening. They will need to be given as much information as they desire in a way they can understand and leaflets can help with this. Many units have leaflets for each therapy with tables for dosing and monitoring, like those above, so the patient can take charge of their own care. Despite this many patients are not able or not willing to play an active role in managing their disease and we must always be sensitive to this. Perhaps the most important piece of information patients can be given is a telephone number with your secretary's contact details on it in case of concerns.

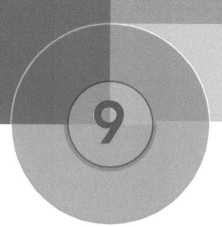

Advanced therapies and future treatments

While conventional immunosuppressants are used to partially poison a patient by disturbing vast swathes of immune function, but only by a selected amount, advanced therapies started to emerge that could affect a specific portion of the inflammatory cascade in the form of monoclonal antibodies. This kind of treatment is called 'biologic' therapy as it implies using the natural biology of the body to effect change rather than work against the entire machine – to disguise spies as civil servants who infiltrate an enemy government agency and alter the paperwork to open the border rather than attack the organised opposition full on. An example of this which ophthalmologists stand a better chance of understanding is the ubiquitous use of anti-vascular endothelial growth factor (VEGF) therapy for choroidal neovascular membranes in almost every eye department in the world. Aflibercept or ranibizumab both have dramatic effects on calming bleeding in age-related macular degeneration which a broad-spectrum equivalent such as a steroid could never achieve, and with fewer side effects by far. The field of biologic therapy is new and exciting and new drugs are being developed that are full of potential in the field of uveitis as well as medical retina. Sticking with the military metaphor it is as if the front line in the fight against uveitis had stabilised into slow trench warfare using steroids and conventional immunosuppressants but the development of biologics is akin to a flanking manoeuvre which has unexpectedly resulted in our troops advancing through mile upon mile of open countryside liberating villages with no real sign of the enemy. It is an exciting time.

These medications were developed for use in rheumatology first and as things stand now, with a few notable exceptions, rheumatologists are still their masters with regards to inflammatory eye disease. Almost universally ophthalmologists do not prescribe or monitor biologic therapies for uveitis and our role is to recognise which patients could benefit and to send them to our rheumatology colleagues to do the needful. These medications delivered systemically are powerful and side effects and interactions can affect almost any part of the body, such that for now eye departments are not geared to take over controlling these medications. On top of this the funding system in the United Kingdom is such that it would be a nightmare if we had to organise our own biologic services and any attempt to transfer this responsibility to us should be resisted at all costs, unless your unit is very large or you have a special research interest. For this reason we do not go into detail on how to monitor these medications here. There are two main issues that concern us as ophthalmologists:

1. How do we know which patients to send for biologic therapy?
2. What are the various types of biologic therapy currently available?

It is important to know the answer to the second question as well as the first as we need to keep up to date with developments to properly liaise with the rheumatology team. It must also be remembered that these medications are eye wateringly expensive at the moment compared with traditional treatment so being specific and exact with our referral increases the chance that for the patient's sake the funding gets approved. Biologic therapies are still immunosuppressants of course, so the advice in Chapter 8 concerning tuberculosis (TB) and varicella zoster virus (VZV) still stands.

HOW DO WE KNOW WHICH PATIENTS TO SEND FOR BIOLOGIC THERAPY?

This is actually an easier question to answer than it first appears. If it is regarded that this therapy is selectively powerful with fewer side effects but is very expensive the groups that it will benefit the most will be obvious. First in line will be children with juvenile idiopathic arthritis (JIA) as preventing side effects in this young group is vital to their long-term vision and general health. Another group includes those with conditions that traditionally require heavy systemic immunosuppression such as Behçet's disease, where an early referral to a rheumatologist for biologic therapy will save time and sight. The third group consists of patients with severe uveitis of any aetiology who have gone through the conventional algorithm of oral steroids and a steroid-sparing agent or even two but the disease for whatever reason is not tamed and the patient continues to deteriorate even though their body is being poisoned with drugs. In certain parts of the country there may be a fourth group consisting of adults with milder uveitis who could use standard immunosuppression, but whose knowledge of Google, angry letter writing skills and inability to perceive the nature of a socialist healthcare system such as the National Health Service (NHS) results in a belief that they are entitled to biologic therapy. Biologics can be regarded perhaps as a steroid sparing agent as they are given to reduce dependency on other more toxic drugs.

WHAT ARE THE VARIOUS TYPES OF BIOLOGIC THERAPY CURRENTLY AVAILABLE?

There are four main categories of biologic: TNF-α blockers, anti-lymphocyte antibodies, interleukin receptor blockers and interferons. It takes a working knowledge of immunology to understand what these terms mean let alone how the actual drugs work and as ophthalmologists generally do not understand in any detail the function of the immune system it is better to use them as labels for the medications for now. This is one further reason why rheumatologists and immunologists are right to keep hold of the responsibility for prescribing and monitoring biologic use.

TNF-α BLOCKERS

TNF stands for tumour necrosis factor which is a cytokine produced by T helper cells and plays a vital role in the inflammatory cascade that sets itself up to cause ocular inflammation. Infliximab was previously the most well-known and well-used TNF-α blocker but has lost its position now to **adalimumab (Humira)**. It is more effective than infliximab, has fewer side effects and is administered via a subcutaneous injection given every 2 weeks in the same manner as insulin, as opposed to the intravenous administration of infliximab. One of the other problems with infliximab is that, over time, many patients develop antibodies to the drug (anti-TNF antibodies), with a consequent decline in efficacy. This is because part of the monoclonal antibody is derived from a mouse antibody. Adalimumab is fully humanised, so the development of antibodies to the drug, while still possible, is much rarer.

Adalimumab can be given at home though there is still a monitoring system needed to prevent serious complications. Adalimumab is most commonly used for the treatment of JIA and Behçet's disease with a possible role to play for first-line treatment of severe Behçet's disease. It is likely the adalimumab will be our most commonly used biological in uveitis for some years to come. This is partly because it is one of the few drugs that has been rigorously evaluated as part of a randomised control trial against placebo (the VISUAL I and VISUAL II trials). These landmark trials showed that the drug significantly reduced the risk of flare-up compared to placebo in active uveitis (the VISUAL I study). In addition, the drug was efficacious in allowing a successful steroid taper in those patients with inactive uveitis (the VISUAL II study).

Etanercept (Enbrel) is a less-effective anti-TNF agent. It only binds to soluble TNF – i.e. free floating plasma TNF rather than the TNF receptor on the cell membrane. Although used by rheumatologists for conditions such as ankylosing spondylitis it is generally ineffective in uveitis, and indeed may even cause uveitis. As a consequence it generally has no role for the uveitis specialist.

Golimumab (Simponi) is a newer biologic that is again delivered subcutaneously but at a reduced frequency of once a month. It has been used to control JIA and severe HLA-B27 uveitis although for now in the TNF-α blocking category adalimumab is still all powerful. There are other such medications in existence but they are not used for treating uveitis so will not be mentioned here.

Though there is much positivity here a word of caution must also be noted. As with many drugs, there are side effects and all these TNF-α blockers have been associated with the unmasking of latent tuberculosis and the development of demyelinating disease. There are also reports that the medications in this class can, in rare cases, actually cause uveitis so this must also be borne in mind if commencement of therapy results in an exacerbation rather than an improvement of inflammatory activity.

ANTI-LYMPHOCYTE ANTIBODIES

These medications work by inhibiting B-cell function or T-cell function, of which we will look at the former first. The drugs in this category work by selectively inhibiting B-cell function by causing them to self-destruct by apoptosis. It might be supposed that processes dependent on T cells might be left unaffected but the fact that these are also affected shows how complicated the immune system is. Of all the medications in this class **rituximab (MabThera)** is the most famous. It is an intravenous infusion that is a lot stronger than the anti-TNF medications as only two doses separated by 2 weeks can be sufficient, although it can be repeated after 6 months or more. Its strength is also its greatest weakness and as it is the equivalent of detonating a nuclear bomb inside the immune system all conventional immunosuppressants plus the anti-TNF drugs must have been tried first. It is generally reserved for severe diseases such as Behçet's disease, severe refractory JIA and granulomatosis with polyangiitis (Wegener's disease) with scleritis as well as idiopathic scleritis that has not responded to conventional therapy. Deaths have been reported following its use.

Whilst rituximab acts against B cells, **abatacept (Orencia)** is a T-cell inhibitor and again is an intravenous infusion regarded as a bit of a nuclear option for treating children with JIA who have not responded to conventional therapy plus anti-TNF drugs. Data published so far indicate it is safer than rituximab though it is very far away from being first-line treatment. There are other medications in this class but they are so rarely used in uveitis that they do not warrant a mention here.

INTERLEUKIN RECEPTOR BLOCKERS

Interleukins, as the name suggests, are cytokines that transmit messages between white cells; T cells in particular. **Daclizumab (Zinbryta, and formerly the discontinued Zenapax)** is the most widely known blocker available and specifically blocks IL-2 receptors, not that this information is useful in the slightest to the vast majority of ophthalmologists. It is given via intravenous infusion, or sometimes subcutaneously. It is currently only licensed for use in relapsing multiple sclerosis (MS). It has been tried in uncontrolled single-centre studies in diverse conditions varying from Vogt–Koyanagi–Harada (VKH) disease, birdshot, JIA, and Behçet's disease, and appears to show some efficacy in most of these conditions with the exception of Behçet's disease.

Another drug that inhibits IL-6 receptors is called **tocilizumab (Actemra)**. This is a humanised monoclonal antibody directed against the IL-6 receptor which is administered by intravenous infusion. It is approved for treatment of rheumatoid arthritis and JIA. Small studies have shown that it can be efficacious in treating chronic uveitic macular oedema which is refractory to conventional therapy such as steroids, immunosuppressives and even other biologics such as anti-TNF therapy. It has been used to treat uveitic macular oedema in JIA, Behçet's, and birdshot. Curiously, and rather paradoxically, while it may be effective in treating macular oedema, it does not always control other aspects of inflammation, for example anterior uveitis or vitritis, in the same eye.

INTERFERONS

The interleukin receptor blockers above function by blocking some signals from getting through but the interferons work by mimicking the signal in order to stimulate certain other parts of the immune system. As the interferons work by actually stimulating the immune system symptoms such as a cold or flu are universal with their use. There are many interferons used for many medical reasons but the only uveitis condition that has been successfully shown to be positively influenced by this is Behçet disease after subcutaneous **interferon-alpha (Intron A)** administration. Although efficacious, its popularity has been limited by the side effects listed above, as well as psychological ill effects such as depression.

FINAL WORD ON BIOLOGIC THERAPIES

This entire group of medications is new, exciting and has all the potential of becoming a major game changer in treating uveitis, once mastered. We are living in a time equivalent to shortly after electricity was discovered, where the potential is there for all to see but while work on a light bulb and other wondrous devices is coming on apace there are still tests being undertaken on whether electricity cures criminal tendencies or ageing, and the mysterious new technology is still not tamed enough such that generators explode from time to time or the wiring burns out due to excessive current flow. Perhaps one day uveitis will be easily managed by an injection given by the patient at home and we will all wonder at the toxicity of some of the medications we used to administer. At this stage we simply do not know where the future will lead us but what is certain is that change is so rapid and exciting that of all the chapters in this book this will be the one that becomes redundant fastest.

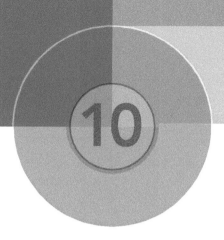

The moral ophthalmologist

10

I attended a course in London at a famous eye hospital, and as is customary with such courses there was an evening of drinks and canapes included so the delegates and lecturers could get to know each other. To my delight a famous hero of uveitis was present and over some slightly sour wine I attempted to tell him my theory of the recent advances in uveitis being akin to the Wild West of America being slowly settled, roads and railways built and eventually counties and states organised so that slowly piece by piece order was being brought to disorder. I emphasised the fact that for now there was still much disagreement among the most influential people in the specialty about where the borders should run as well as the best locations for the main transport routes to California. He drank his wine and dismissed my theory out of hand. 'It's already settled' he said. 'Everybody knows what the eventual shape of the nation will be in your example. The only thing keeping uveitis specialists from making real gains is the arrogance of so many of the key people in thinking that their way is the only way while all along there is a right way of doing things under all the egotism'. This statement intrigued me and I asked him that if there was indeed a 'correct' way of doing things what was that way? He looked down at his wine glass for a second, hesitated and looked directly at me. 'My way' he said, and laughed.

This book is not a textbook. This book is not an in-depth analysis of all the latest research. This book does not contain all the information needed to work in a uveitis clinic. What this book is meant to do is to explain the thousands of simple things that are not told to new ophthalmologists entering the field of uveitis and to give them a grounding so that if more information is needed they are better equipped to be able to find it more easily. The algorithms, doses, classifications and drugs mentioned are not absolute and many eye units would do things differently. They are however safe and provide a way of getting by until local policies are explained and understood. It is not uncommon for fellows at some of the greatest eye hospitals in the world to go through an entire year of experience without truly understanding the aims and objectives of treatment, though they might learn tens of thousands of less important facts. This book represents the travel writings of a person who has travelled across the unorganised lands of the American West pointing out various geographical features while making some comment about how the senators in Washington think in future the land will be divided and where the new state capitals will likely be. Both of us hope you find it accessible and useful.

Once a basic knowledge of uveitis is gained and the basic aims and treatments of therapy understood you will find yourselves immediately propelled to the status of relative experts in the field. This is because ophthalmologists are scared of uveitis and scared of the toxic treatments that are used and for now at least the uveitis specialist is regarded as a witch doctor or shaman that appears out of nowhere spouting long words and casting spells before disappearing in a cloud of blue smoke. Paediatric ophthalmologists with their understanding of the rarefied language of orthoptics are the only speciality that comes close to ours with regards mystery and impenetrability. Although it is very impressive to pull a diagnosis seemingly out of thin air we must aim to show our working. Like petrified villagers trainees will be in awe of uveitis but not attempt to understand it if we purposefully disguise the logical and scientific process at the heart of what we are doing. It is good for the patient, for the trainee and for the speciality if it is made more accessible and all efforts should be made to explain how diagnoses are reached and why treatments follow the patterns that they do. Otherwise we will not be properly training the next generation beyond inducing the birth of a form of cargo cult, where Indonesian jungle dwellers during the Second World War built mock runways and control towers in the erroneous belief that it was this peculiar form of worship that resulted in the heavenly delivery of airborne cargo. They had misunderstood the basics. When an ophthalmologist sees a patient with an inflamed eye and picks up a blood form ticking every single box present while remembering he saw the boss order a few blood tests in just this sort of circumstance a few weeks ago, we are not spreading enlightenment. The aeroplanes with their precious cargo will not come.

Hippocrates made the duty of training new doctors part of his oath. As we were ourselves trained so we should train others. When a colleague comes to us with a case of what might seem like an easily managed uveitis it is easy to forget that to them this case might be incredibly worrying. This colleague might be a fellow consultant as well as a trainee, or even a doctor from another specialty. Unless there are specific reasons not to do so always try and see the patient. Go with the doctor and examine the patient for yourself. Explain why you think the way you do and if it is a colleague asking for help offer to take over care of the patient. It is not becoming to wait until formally asked; if your colleague in fact wants to retain the patient under their care then they will be pleased at your offer and happy that there is a source of support available should he run into trouble.

Ivory towers need not be very tall. If you are becoming frustrated at the numbers of simple anterior uveitis cases referred to your clinic it is possible that further training of eye casualty staff or constructing a document with an algorithm with appropriate treatment regimens might solve the problem. It is sadly not that uncommon to adopt the sour grumpy face tactic in a bid to deter people from asking you about cases. Perhaps you are too busy, have a meeting to get to or are simply tired after a long day, but within each eye department trainees will rapidly get to know who is approachable and who is not. The Parable of the Talents tells a story whereby three servants are given varying amounts of money, with two investing it and making more money and the youngest burying it in the ground to keep it safe. The master upon his return is furious and takes the buried money away from the servant who had kept it hidden and gives it to the other two – 'For whoever has, to him shall be given and he shall have more abundance. But whoever does not have, from him shall be taken away even that which he has'. While strictly speaking this tale was told in relation to knowledge of the Kingdom of Heaven it has been applied to many situations over the two millennia since it was first spoken and uveitis is no exception. Essentially the knowledge and experience of a uveitis consultant who is friendly and approachable and works through problems with those who come to ask advice will blossom and grow while the knowledge of the uveitis specialist who discourages anyone from asking for help and shuts themselves off from the department around them will wither and die.

There is no shame in admitting that you do not know the answer. In fact it is common that the answer will not be immediately obvious. It is a sign of maturity that a person will admit to not knowing rather than attempt to befuddle others with distractions. Prof. Bird, Mr. Pavesio and Prof. Lightman all of Moorfields fame will admit if they do not immediately know the answer to a clinical problem and they will do so happily. I have no doubt that the other great experts in the world do the same. What sets them apart however is that they all have a system of reaching the truth that is logical and consistent, and this is something that is aided by and grows with experience, by accepting cases and seeing things through to the end. Very few diagnoses are spot diagnoses. As an ophthalmologist in training it is vital you make a note of all interesting cases or those in which the diagnosis is uncertain and follow them through to the end. There are always lessons to be learnt. Presenting interesting cases to your colleagues will help you as much as it will them. All of this advice applies to all ophthalmologists in all positions. We never stop being students, and we should never forget that.

Index